Sleep Medicine and the Evolution of Contemporary Sleep Pharmacotherapy

Edited by Denis Larrivee

Published in London, United Kingdom

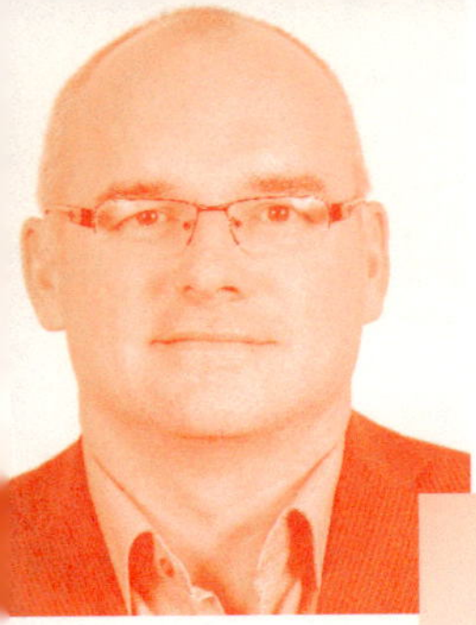
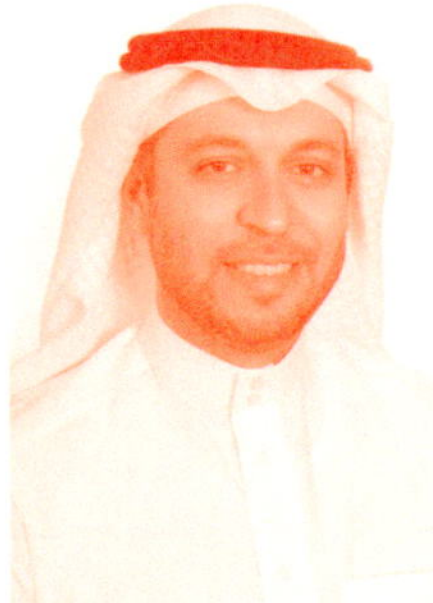
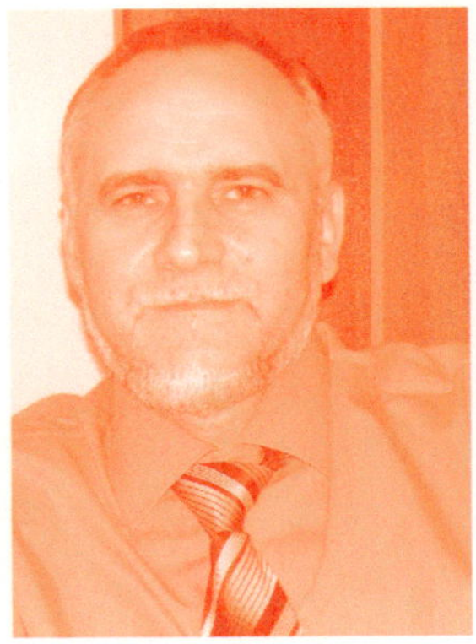
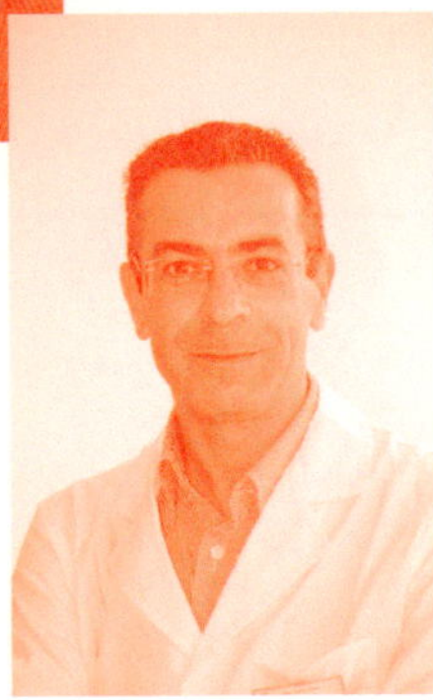
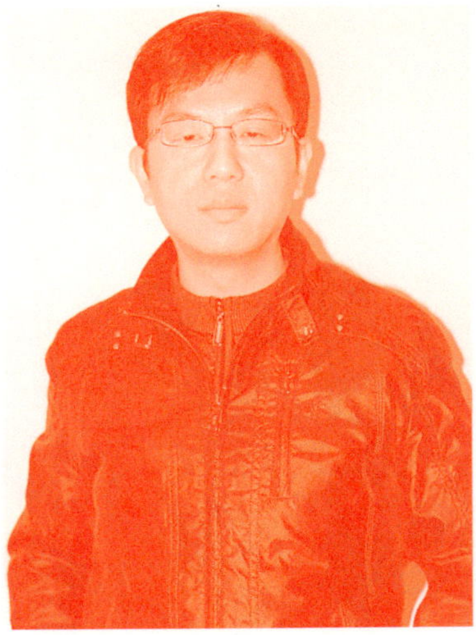
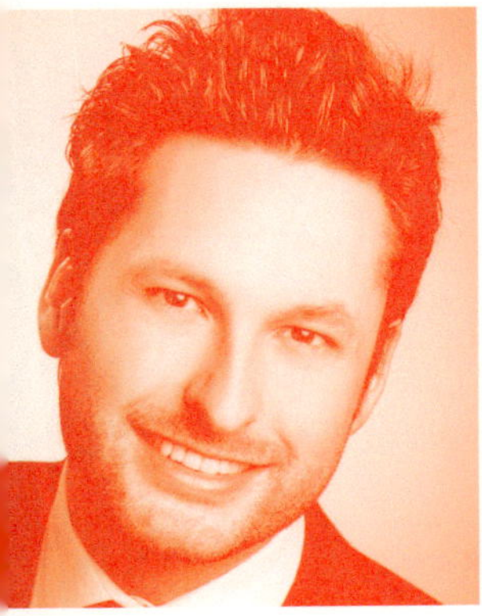
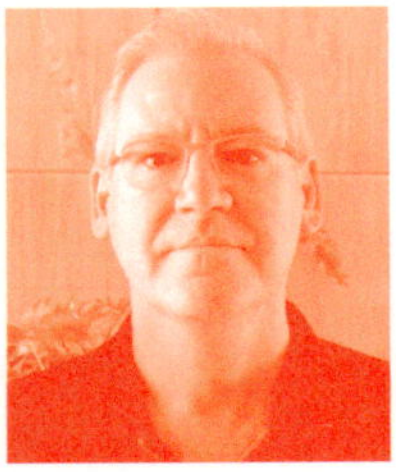

IntechOpen

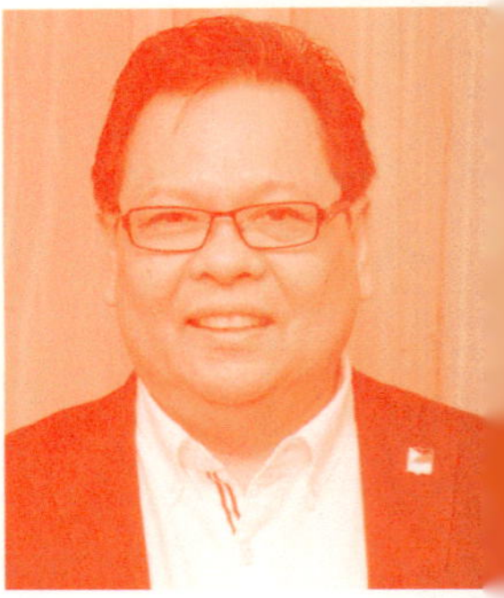
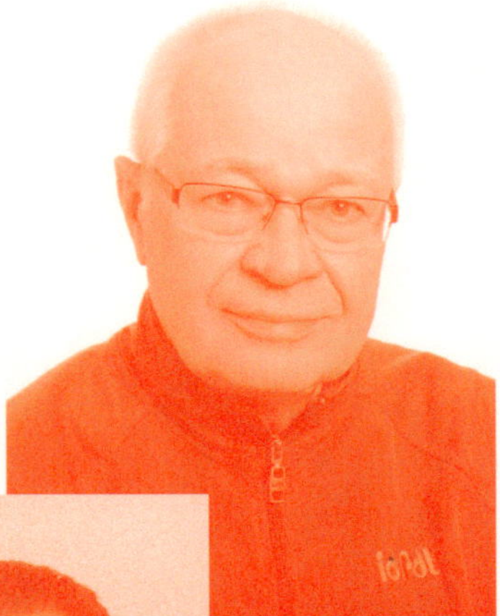
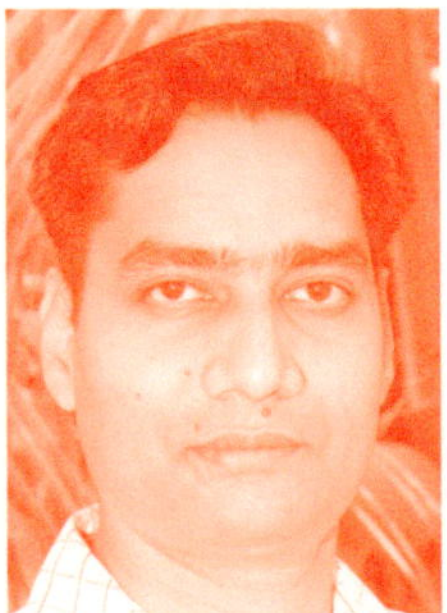
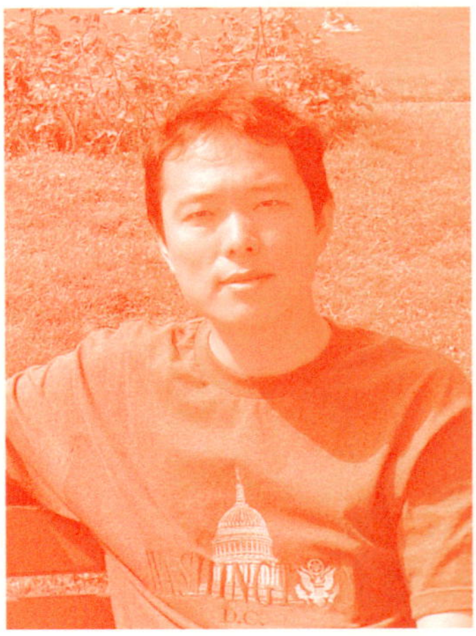
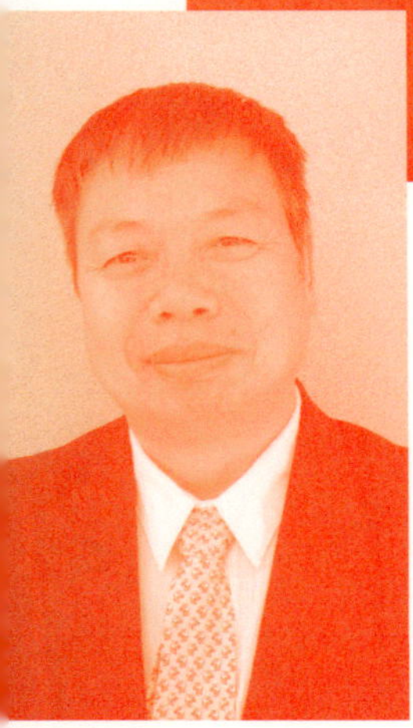
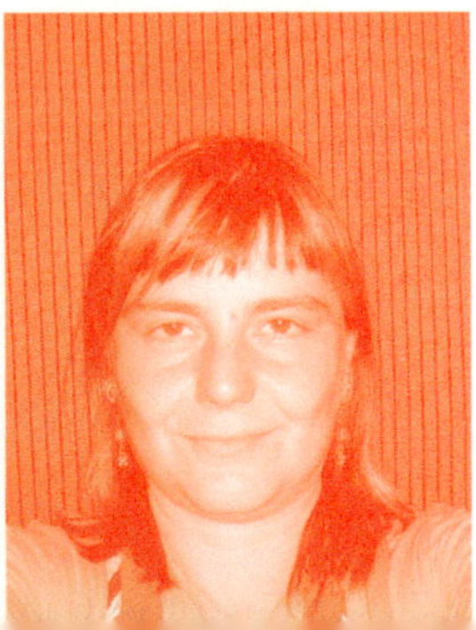

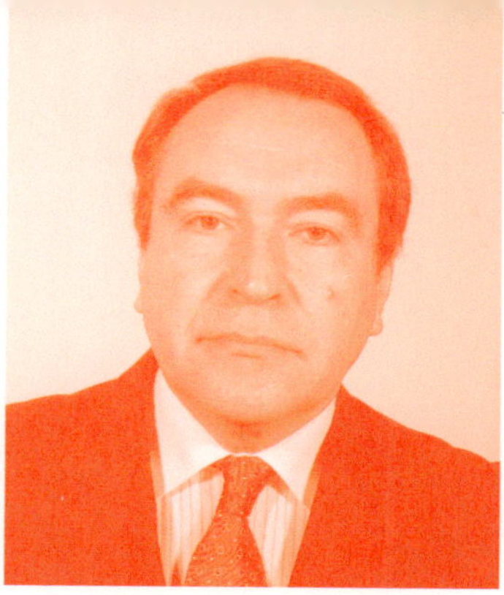
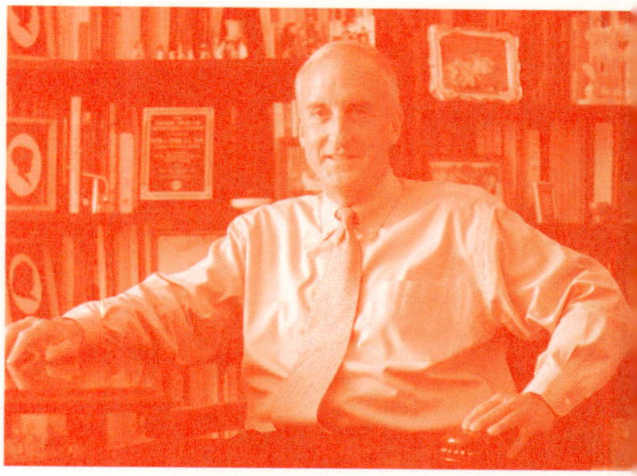
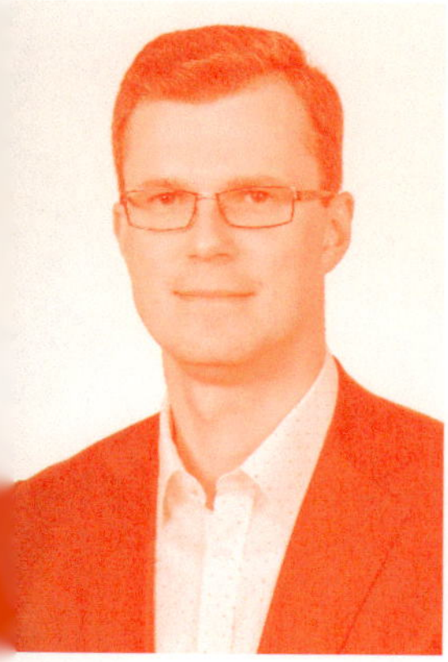
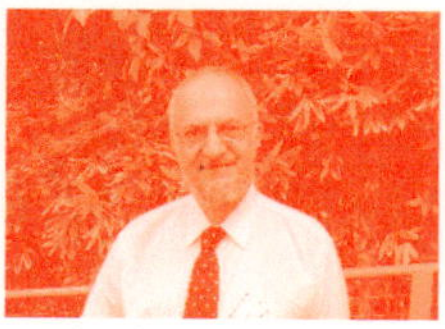
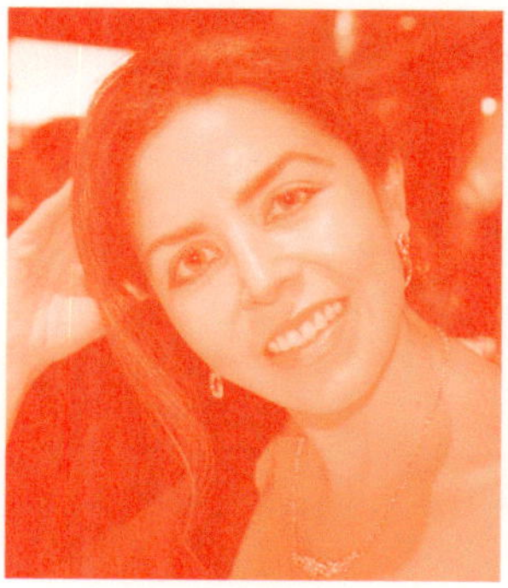

Supporting open minds since 2005

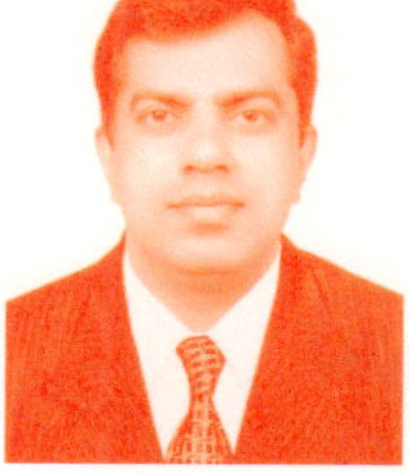
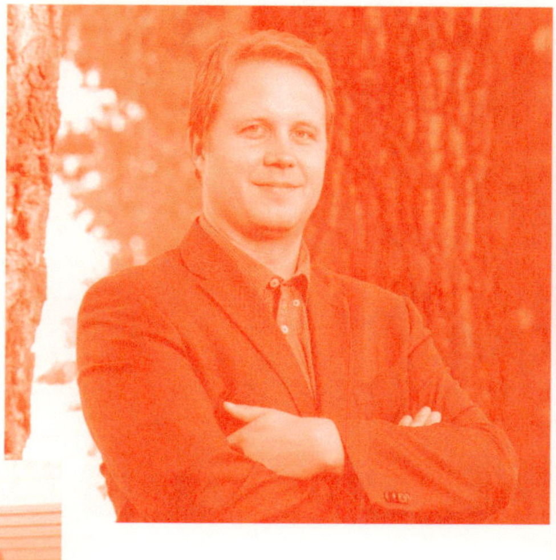
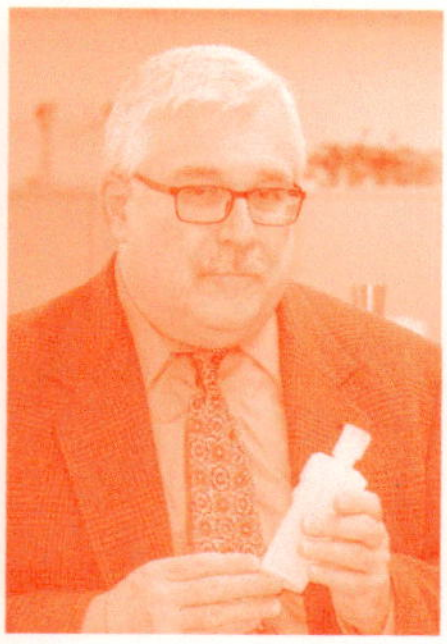
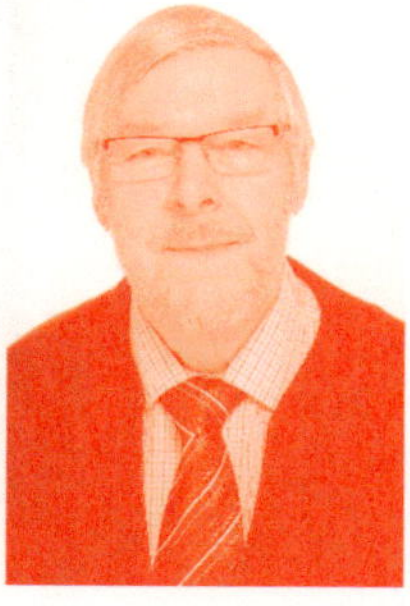
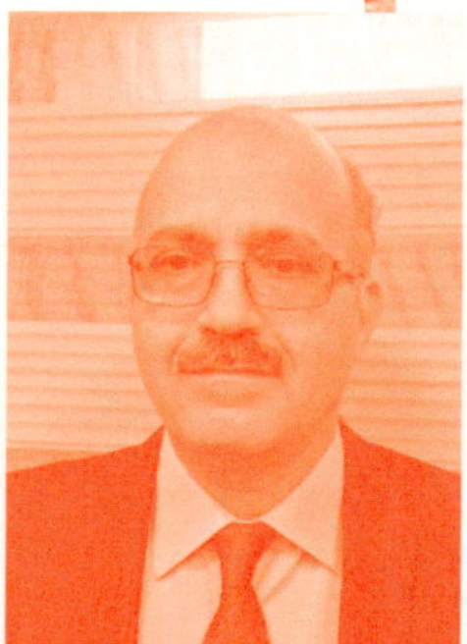
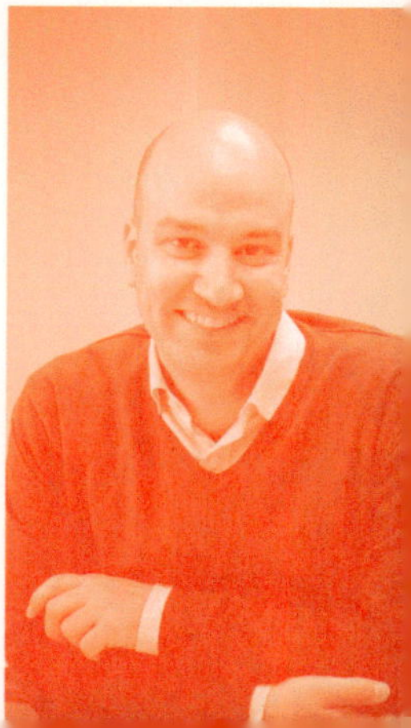
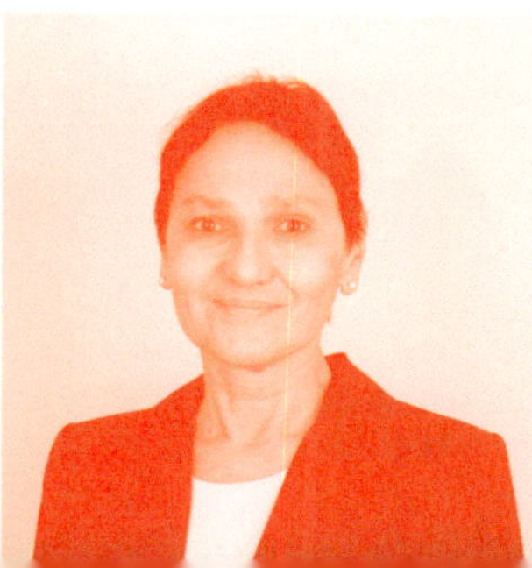

Sleep Medicine and the Evolution of Contemporary Sleep Pharmacotherapy
http://dx.doi.org/10.5772/intechopen.91536
Edited by Denis Larrivee

Contributors
Ajay Sampat, Armand Ryden, Kristina Keller, Stefan Lakämper, Murat Kayabekir, Juan José Ortega-Albás, Raquel López García, Alfonso Martínez Martínez, Sonia Carratalá Monfort, Juan Antonio Royo Prats, Laura Albiol Varela, Patricia Ortega Gabás, Gregory S. Carter, Mihaela Pantea, Teodor Traistaru, Ana Maria Cristina Țâncu, Marina Imre, Patrizia Moretti, Lucia Gonfia, Giulia Menculini, Bing Tang, Denis Larrivee

First published in London, United Kingdom, 2022 by IntechOpen
IntechOpen is the global imprint of INTECHOPEN LIMITED, registered in England and Wales, registration number: 11086078, 5 Princes Gate Court, London, SW7 2QJ, United Kingdom
Printed in Croatia

British Library Cataloguing-in-Publication Data
A catalogue record for this book is available from the British Library

Additional hard and PDF copies can be obtained from orders@intechopen.com

Sleep Medicine and the Evolution of Contemporary Sleep Pharmacotherapy
Edited by Denis Larrivee
p. cm.
Print ISBN 978-1-83969-821-7
Online ISBN 978-1-83969-822-4
eBook (PDF) ISBN 978-1-83969-823-1

For EU product safety concerns:
IN TECH d.o.o., Prolaz Marije Krucifikse Kozulić 3, 51000 Rijeka, Croatia, info@intechopen.com or visit our website at intechopen.com.

Meet the editor

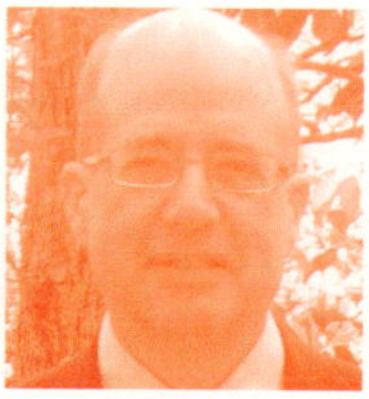

Dr. Denis Larrivee is a visiting scholar at the Mind and Brain Institute, Las Vegas; University of Navarra Medical School, Spain; and Loyola University Chicago. He has held professorships at Weill Cornell University Medical College, NYC, and Purdue University, Indiana. A former fellow at Yale University's Medical School Dr. Larrivee received the Association for Research in Vision and Ophthalmology's first-place award for studies on photoreceptor degenerative and developmental mechanisms. He is the chief editor of several medical and scientific texts, including topics on brain- computer interfacing, Alzheimer's disease, neuromodulation and neurostimulation procedures, neuroethics, and sleep pharmacotherapies. He is an editorial board member of the journals *Annals of Neurology and Neurological Sciences* and *EC Neurology*. An International Neuroethics Society Expert he is the author of more than ninety papers and book chapters in such varied journals/venues as *Neurology and Neurological Sciences, Journal of Neuroscience, Journal of Religion and Mental Health*, and *IEEE Explore*. In 2018 he was a finalist in the international Joseph Ratzinger Expanded Reason Award sponsored by the Francis Vittorio University of Madrid.

Contents

Preface

Changes in daily living circumstances over several decades have significantly affected sleep quality, propelling two revolutions in health care: a treatment revolution, which has been directed to the care of sleep disturbances, chiefly through pharmacological methods, and a research revolution, which has produced a novel understanding of the role of sleep in cognition. High-paced social and employment practices, for instance, have notably combined to make insomnia a major dysfunction affecting both physical and mental health, with nearly 30%–40% of the adult population suffering from its mild to severe forms.

The need to treat insomnia and other sleep disorders has been the stimulus for developing pharmacologic interventions that, historically, have pursued an empiric approach. This approach has yielded drug candidates capable of alleviating sleep disturbances, but often with accompanying undesirable effects. Benzodiazepines, the first group of sleep medications developed, exhibited significant adverse effects like cognitive and psychomotor impairment, anterograde amnesia, next-day hangover, and rebound insomnia. Because of these adverse effects, the use of benzodiazepines for treatment of insomnia became controversial. In their place the non-benzodiazepine drugs like zolpidem, zaleplon, and zopiclone that followed all had high affinity and selectivity for the a1-subunit of the GABAA receptor complex, which improved sleep maintenance shortly after administration but lost this effect, however, at later sleep stages. These drugs too had adverse effects, which included daytime drowsiness, dizziness, headache, and nausea. In like manner, empirical approaches have yielded other drug candidates such as the orexin blockers with their own suite of advantages and disadvantages. Following this empirical progression has thus altogether yielded an extensive, proliferating, and somewhat bewildering variety of sleep medications, with the current pharmacopeia now exhibiting a broad range of biological properties affecting sleep.

Coincident with the revolution in sleep pharmacotherapy there has been a parallel revolution in the understanding of the nature of sleep. While motivated chiefly by the health needs of increasing numbers of individuals suffering sleep disturbances, the study of the physical reality of sleep also presented itself as a strikingly interesting, universal feature of cognition. All known mammalian species notably exhibit sleep. This universal physical feature led to numerous studies that attempted to explain sleep's biophysical basis. Dominating the hypothetical landscape was the fact that sleep's defining feature entailed a sensory disconnection from afferent input. Addressing the why and how of this feature has now yielded key insights into the nature of sleep with a growing body of data coalescing around several models. These models point to a global influence in the modulation of the neuroplastic events of cognition and thus of an influence likely to be exerted on neurological functions throughout the brain.

The text presented here is a recognition of these twin revolutions, which have been driven by the need to address a common and increasingly prevalent class of health and social impairments.

This text, however, is also a recognition that the revolutions in pharmacological medications and in the understanding of the physical basis of sleep are windows into a broader view of systemic dysfunction within the brain and so of the cross-cutting relevance of sleep for the practice of medicine in numerous neurological domains. This is to say that both the understanding of sleep and the methodology evolved for its treatment have reached a point of synergy that represents a plateau with broader implications for therapeutic intervention in cognitive dysfunction.

Consistent with this view, several studies have reported that sleep and psychiatric disorders are comorbid, such as depression or anxiety, suggesting that sleep disturbances may constitute etiological factors contributing to psychiatric impairments. Indeed, the identification of comorbidities ranging from psychoses and addiction to neurological dysfunction and the like is a significant indicator that processes like sleep that operate on global scales are likely to have wide-ranging functional effects.

Accordingly, this book presents an up-to-date portrait of these revolutions, demonstrating the success achieved in pharmacological therapy and the insights acquired through research exploration. However, the text is also intended to link these findings to efforts to chart a trajectory that will reveal the cross-cutting relevance of sleep pharmacotherapy not only for the medical management of its disorders but also for the practice of medicine in a wider range of neurological issues.

To present these themes, the chapters are anchored by an introductory discussion on the contemporary understanding of the biological and physical basis of sleep and the implications that this understanding has about cognition and the physiological mechanisms that are themselves affected by sleep. These mechanisms are then discussed from the vantage of pharmacological tools that are capable of modulating sleep events and therapeutically resolving its disturbances. A final section considers the therapeutic terrain beyond sleep disturbances, the neurological domain of sleep-induced, system dysfunction.

Current models of sleep situate it within the sphere of biophysical phenomena and often characterize it as adhering strictly to fundamental physical principles. The bodily processes that govern sleep and establish its rhythms are therefore themselves constrained to accommodate these principles within the architecture shaping sleep behavior. The biochemical medium underpinning this behavior is taken up in Chapter 2. Included in its discussion is a comprehensive compendium of the many small regulatory molecules involved in sleep and circadian rhythms. Their roles in brain systems physiology, hypothalamic and pituitary hormone influences in sleep, neuropharmacological agents, and changes during psychiatric disease are presented, an organization that assists not only in relating their molecular contribution to brain systems physiology but that is also helpful in understanding how they are likely to interact with each other in normal and pathological circumstances.

The disruption of sleep regulatory mechanisms constitutes the most visible aspect of sleep disturbances, their biochemical, electrophysiological, and behavioral features having motivated the progressive evolution in the present pharmacopeia. Chapters 3 and 4 consider two well-known symptomatic consequences of failures in sleep regulation mechanisms: narcolepsy and the parasomnias.

Narcolepsy is one of the most common causes of chronic sleepiness, occurring in nearly one of every 2000 individuals with significant impact on quality of life and employment. Chapter 3 by Jose et al. highlights current pharmacotherapeutic practice for narcolepsy, which has a stated intention of managing but not curing the disease. Its discussion addresses first- and second-line treatments, combined therapies, kinetic profiles, and other details of the chief pharmaceuticals now available for medical management of narcolepsy, a compendium that should be useful for the physician not frequently accustomed to treating this class of patients. Parasomnias are unusual motor and/or behavioral events that occur while falling asleep, during sleep, or arousal, which may appear in rapid eye movement (REM) or non-REM (NREM) phases of sleep. In pediatric populations, they can be highly prevalent, as in NREM parasomnias, attaining nearly 40%. Chapter 4 by Carter reviews the principal parasomnia classes, sleep-related movement disorders, REM and NREM parasomnias, and arousal disorders, their symptomatology, and contraindications. The discussion considers not only pharmacokinetics, bioavailability, receptor physiology, and system influences, but also provides a wealth of physical molecular features (e.g., the presence of single vs double rings, receptor binding site interactions, affinity constants, etc.) that distinguishes compound classes as considered effects of their biological action. Included are such major players as the benzodiazepines; melatonin; antidepressants; alpha delta, voltage-gated, calcium channel blockers; dopamine agonists; and opioids.

Beyond the symptomatic expression of direct regulatory dysfunction, sleep disturbances encompass ancillary symptoms whose modalities significantly, but indirectly, impinge on secondary systemic wellbeing. Chapters 5 and 6 consider the special case of apnea, with Chapter 5 exploring the significance of a risk indicator in a previously unassessed, cultural setting, Taiwan, and Chapter 6 the diagnostic breadth offered by supplementary disciplines.

Chapter 5 explores the link between snoring and obstructive sleep apnea (OSA), a predisposing risk factor causative for cardiovascular disease and associated dysfunctions, including hypertension, arrhythmia, coronary heart disease, and stroke. The author's focus on variables relating to altered suprachiasmatic nuclear function is useful for relating apnea to a neurological basis. Chapter 6 takes up the symbiotic and growing intersection between the medical dental disciplines and the clinical specialties associated with sleep and disorders of the upper respiratory airway, notably OSA. As the authors state, the intersection between disciplines is comprehensive, including diagnosis, therapy, and medical management. This is a significant evolution in two previously disparate approaches to upper airway dysfunction affecting normal health.

The remaining three chapters chart territory that moves beyond sleep processes themselves to the effects of sleep dysfunction in the public health arena (Chapter 7), circadian rhythmic alterations and their effects on health and wellbeing (Chapter 8), and influences on maternal wellbeing and bodily development during pregnancy (Chapter 9).

Chapter 7 takes up the very significant issue of the difficult balance required for navigation between threats to traffic safety and sleep dysfunctions harmful to drivers. Compounding this difficult balance has been the proliferation in pharmacological products affecting sleep, often obtained in over-the-counter formulations. The authors of the chapter address this situation by discussing the legal and medical framework that has evolved in Switzerland for preserving public safety while also providing for personal medical needs.

The lack of synchrony between an individual's internal, circadian rhythm and locally experienced, environmental time can significantly impair quality of life. Chapter 8 identifies the chief rhythmic dysfunctions that are observed clinically, provides a diagnostic guide for the screening and evaluating of these dysfunctions, and introduces basic treatment strategies that can be applied by non-sleep medicine clinicians. The chapter also discusses the effect of these daily rhythm disorders on the functioning of other organ systems.

Sleep and circadian rhythm dysfunction can also impact development by affecting pregnancy symptoms and outcomes, as discussed in Chapter 9. A widely replicated observation, for example, is the change seen in the Pittsburgh Sleep Quality Index. Maternal effects introduced by these dysfunctions can extend to the foetus, who lacks intrinsic circadian mechanisms and must depend on their maternal origin to function. Small birth weights, growth retardation, and the subsequent evolution of high blood pressure are among the significant effects on secondary systems that are experienced by the foetus. Chapter 9 discusses the unique medical management of sleep required for disorders during pregnancy, which is complicated by the potential for harm to the foetus from pharmaceutical compounds used to treat sleep dysfunction of the mother, as well as numerous secondary effects occurring in both mother and child.

It is my hope that readers of this text will come to appreciate the medical significance of sleep therapy not solely for treating sleep disturbances but also for the care of other neurological symptoms for which the influence of sleep is only beginning to be understood.

Denis Larrivee
Mind and Brain Institute,
University of Navarra Medical School,
Pamplona, Spain

Department of Arts and Sciences,
Loyola University Chicago,
Chicago, USA

Section 1

Sleep and Its Systemic Association

Chapter 1

Introductory Chapter: The Promise of Sleep Pharmacotherapy - Healing Systems Level Dysfunction

Denis Larrivee

1. Introduction

Perhaps no behavioral feature is more evident and more widely distributed, nor more sought after than sleep. Yet, it is for its distinctiveness that sleep has often seemed at odds with daily needs, where attention and responsivity are critical to survival. Its presence, therefore, reveals the existence of some undetermined physical need, which no other mechanism can physically respond to.

Given the prominence and regularity of sleep, this physical need, and the physiological mechanisms used to satisfy it, can be expected to exert an influence on many bodily processes. Indeed, the events of sleep are now known to affect a broad number of fundamental bodily systems that may be enhanced or diminished in parallel with sleep phases. Sleep or circadian-related influences, for example, have been documented for autonomic function [1], hormone secretion/core-body temperature rhythm [2], energy production such as glucose metabolism [3], and coordinated motor and immune functions. By extension, disruption of sleep mechanisms can be expected to negatively impact the many processes that are subject to their influence [4].

A growing body of evidence indicates that the events of sleep have their origin in properties of the brain and nervous system circuitry. During NREM sleep, for instance, down states have been shown to be associated with a slowly traveling, oscillation wave that is synchronized throughout the cortex and substantial portions of the subcortex [5]. Transitioning between sleep stages, additionally, involves the modulation of an arousal system that is distributed throughout the brain and that choreographs the shape of sleep architecture. These and many other details imply that the systemic processes affected by sleep are initially affected by a global impact exerted at the level of the brain, which potentially affects such events as developmental regimes of synaptogenesis [6], psychiatric dysfunctions [7], addiction [8], hormonal rhythms [1], and cognitive processes like memory and learning [9].

Those dysfunctional sleep mechanisms that can be linked to secondary systemic dysfunctions offer the intriguing possibility of medically managing and even of therapeutically alleviating such dysfunctions through treatment modalities developed chiefly for sleep disturbances. Drugs that enhance states of sleep, for instance, are also known to alter autonomic physiology, behavior, cognition, and affect [10]. While the complexities of the brain's neurochemistry and circuits mediating

IntechOpen

wakefulness and sleep make the control of the precise physiological mechanisms uncertain, there has been considerable progress in developing medications that are narrowly tailored to various features of sleep, such as rapid sleep onset, minimal hangover, and low abuse potential, among other properties [11]. That is, the current evolution in sleep pharmacotherapy has generated an armamentarium of sufficient precision that it may be redirected to other neural systems. An improving database, moreover, can be expected to further the ability to tailor sleep modulation so as to selectively modulate events directly affected by sleep mechanisms.

An important component of rational therapeutic intervention, nonetheless, clearly also requires a continually improving understanding of the sleep mechanisms themselves [12]. This is to say that only from a knowledge of sleep can the understanding of how it affects other systems be discerned. Accordingly, this chapter will review several leading hypotheses regarding the physical properties that govern sleep mechanisms, the prospects for modulating these properties pharmacologically, and the systemic effects such therapy may have.

2. The universal need for sleep

Each time sleep occurs the ability to appraise the events around us is lost. This interruption of sensorial content represents a definitional and unique feature of sleep, one that distinguishes it from other behavioral states, all of which otherwise retain the ability to promptly respond to stimuli. Although it is unknown why it should be necessary to prevent the brain from receiving input for prolonged intervals, the fact that humans and all other animal species require sleep indicates the existence of a fundamental physical and neural reason for it to occur; that is, sleep serves at least one essential function that cannot be carried out while awake.

One widely acknowledged proposal links this essential function to neuronal properties evoked by centrally directed communication, which involves changes in interneuronal exchange at the level of the synapse. This hypothesis, termed the synaptic homeostasis hypothesis (SHY), privileges the unique ability of the brain to learn from external events of the world that become inscribed through neuroplastic changes in synaptic connections [12]. The SHY hypothesis proposes that these neuroplastic changes entail sensorium-induced increases in synaptic potentiation, which can be visualized electrophysiologically in miniature endplate potentials; that is, there is a *sensorium-induced* increase in synaptic potentiation. Because the extent of potentiation necessarily possesses an upper limit, there is a need to regularly reduce the level of potentiation so that the brain can continue to learn. This readjustment is proposed to occur during sleep.

Hence, sleep is the mechanism that has evolved to account for the cost of the physical events of neuroplasticity, which enable the organism to adapt and survive in a constantly changing environment [13]. When this cost is not accounted for cognitive function is poor. Acute and chronic sleep loss, for example, have pervasive negative effects on performance and many brain functions, including the ability to learn, remember, speak clearly, judge risk, and understand complex information needed for decision making [14]. Post-training "fatigue," for example, the impaired capacity for new learning that follows intense training in a motor or visual task, is restored only by sleep. Physically, therefore, sleep assists in maintaining an overall balance of synaptic strength across brain circuits, which may be conceived as a synaptic renormalization. The hypothesis thus predicts that overall synaptic strength in the brain should not be balanced at all times, but instead should be biased toward a net potentiation during the major wake period and toward a net depression during sleep.

Similar to the SHY hypothesis, the free energy principle of Friston and colleagues hypothesizes that ongoing informational input from the sensorium leads to a rise in the information-related, state variable, entropy [15]. Like potentiation, entropy is a saturable quantity driven by sensorial input that progressively approaches an upper bound. Unlike the potentiation hypothesis, the free energy principle does not postulate a specific period devoted to recovery from synaptic changes. Instead, the brain is proposed to counter the ensuing information accumulation by optimizing behavioral patterns that minimize the need for future change. For instance, inputs that occur together more frequently than would be expected by chance are registered because they suggest regularities in the environment that are predictable. Once these "coincidences" are detected, a neuron communicates them to its target neuron, typically through synaptic strengthening. The effect of registering these "coincidences" thus enables the brain to structure its behavior so as to minimize surprisal and guide the selection of behavioral responses. By such active inferencing [16], the brain comes to reflect the regularities observed in the external world, an organizational arrangement that serves to maximize free energy efficiency.

The free energy principle governing cognition resembles aspects of the SHY hypothesis in providing an explanation for changes in synaptic events that are due to sensorial input and that build on the brain's ability to enable the organism to better confront a continually changing, environmental landscape. Moreover, by staging causal optimization in terms of an entropic cost function, the model accounts for some physical constraints that place an upper bound on synaptic change.

Nonetheless, the free energy principle only indirectly addresses the issue of saturability due to ongoing sensorial novelty, which is inherent in the interactive circumstances of the external world and presumably greatly amplified by the presence of living organisms [17]. This means that the persistence of novel input from the sensorium will continue to generate synaptic reorganization, despite causal inferencing that may diminish the overall level of reorganization. Faced with ongoing novelty, organizational resources of brain synapses can be expected to operate within physical ranges that regularly encounter upper limits under the assumptions of both proposals. Indeed, the observation that all known animal species need to "regularly disconnect" constitutes a strong argument that sensorial novelty is persistent and that its input repeatedly saturates a physical condition that must subsequently be replenished; that is, the brain is "awash" in new experiences for which physical compensation is required. *Hence, while the free energy principle is agnostic with regard to underlying mechanisms that result in saturability, both it and the SHY hypothesis link sleep to ongoing afferent input that modifies the brain's synaptic organization in such a manner as to regularly require renormalization.*

3. Theoretical implications of current sleep models

This conclusion, drawn from two leading proposals that describe sleep mechanisms, has several implications. First – though tautological, existing evidence strongly supports it – observable replenishment mechanisms should entail a sensorial disconnection from the external world and so renormalization should occur during unconsciousness. It has been argued for instance [12] that if the nervous system must acquire information about the environment to survive, such acquisition should be confined to periods of waking rather than during sleep, when neural activity is at least partly disconnected from the external world" [18]. Second, such mechanisms should occur globally; that is, at a minimum, they should be found in all brain domains having sensorial input. Additionally, neuroplastic changes should also affect downstream targeted destinations; that is, rather than modifying only brain regions receiving direct sensorial input, connectivity changes should be distributed across most domains of the brain. Thirdly, renormalization should occur cyclically, a conclusion that is implicit in the first two consequences of these hypotheses.

3.1 Disconnecting from the sensorium

For excitatory synapses, which account for the majority of the synapses in the mammalian brain, the first prediction has received support from molecular, ultrastructural, and electrophysiological measures of synaptic strength [19]. At the molecular level, changes in the strength of excitatory synapses have been shown to involve changes in the surface expression and subunit composition of the glutamatergic AMPA receptors, as well as phosphorylation and other post-translational changes that alter the open probability of these receptors and their ability to remain anchored to the membrane. Surface insertion of GluA1-containing receptors, and the phosphorylation of GluA1 at Ser831 and Ser845 by CaMKII and PKA, particularly, have been correlated with synaptic potentiation.

RNA-seq analysis in the adult mouse frontal cortex, moreover, has revealed a significant overlap of transcripts differentially expressed between acute sleep deprivation and sleep, and transcripts affected by the loss of the transcription factor myocyte enhancer factor 2C (MEF2C) [20]. This study also found a relative dephosphorylation of MEF2C after 6 h of sleep deprivation as compared to sleep, consistent with a wake-related increase in MEF2C transcriptional activity. Additionally, the study observed an increase in the frequency and amplitude of mEPSCs. Altogether, these findings point to a key role for MEF2C in mediating the response to sleep deprivation and the sleep-dependent decline in excitatory synaptic strength. Consistent with this, MEF2 transcriptional activity is activated in response to glutamate release and membrane depolarization, with the main effect of MEF2 activity in postmitotic neurons that of constraining of dendritic spines and excitatory synapses [21]. Many targets of MEF2, additionally, have been shown to be involved in synaptic weakening, including the genes *Arc* and *Homer1a*.

Electrophysiologically, experimental evidence supports distinct physical changes during the wake or sleep periods that are reflected in spontaneous miniature excitatory postsynaptic currents (mEPSCs) in the rodent cortex. By the end of the wakeful period, the amplitude and frequency of mEPSCs increase in the superficial layers of the rat and mouse frontal cortices whereas following recovery sleep they decrease. Ultrastructurally, the increase of the former has been correlated with the synaptic insertion of calcium-permeable AMPA receptors [22]. During sleep, this GluA1 synaptic expression decreases with a corresponding shrinkage of the axon-spine interface.

3.2 The global distribution of sleep mechanisms

The second implication of these proposals is that renormalization should occur globally; that is, if sleep is a consequence of enhanced synaptic strengthening, renormalization should occur in all brain regions where sensorial input causes neuroplastic change.

Current evidence indicates that for this to occur neuronal activity is crucial, especially during NREM sleep, which comprises roughly 80% of all sleep time. New studies show that down selection is, surprisingly, a consequence of spiking activity involving several distinct electrophysiological signatures, including hippocampal sharp waves, ripples, and slow oscillations [23]. Despite a broad consensus that

SWRs are likely candidates for inducing synaptic potentiation, recent studies have shown that SWRs promote synaptic weakening instead [24]. Consistent with these results, closed-loop optogenetic inhibition of SWRs prevents the decline in the slope of hippocampal fEPSPs that normally occurs in sleeping mice. Furthermore, such experimental inhibition reduces firing during the ON/UP states of the slow oscillation and prevents post-sleep improvement in neuroprosthetic learning. The same optogenetic manipulation during the DOWN/OFF periods has no effect, showing that the UP state of the slow oscillation – that is, the activity phase -– is the critical period required for down-selection to occur.

Significantly, sleep-dependent renormalization seems to spare those neurons and/or synapses that are most active during sleep. It is well established, for example, that neurons activated during exploration and learning are preferentially reactivated with a similar sequential pattern of firing during SWRs, while disruption of SWRs impairs memory [25], suggesting that they play an important role in its consolidation.

Organization of sharp waves and ripples appears to be mediated by a distinctive, slow oscillation that features prominently during NREM sleep. The slow oscillation wave originates from the thalamus and cortex and oscillates roughly every second between an UP period of depolarization with spiking and a DOWN/OFF period of hyperpolarization with neuronal silence [26]. During non-REM (NREM) sleep, for instance, neural activity is observed in the EEG as a succession of K-complexes, sleep spindles, and slow waves. This defining feature of NREM sleep occurs more or less in synchrony across all neurons, allowing their pooled activity to be detected at the cortical surface as slow waves. This means that the slow oscillation is a global, synchronized network phenomenon, involving neurons throughout the cortex and, to a lesser degree, neurons in subcortical areas, including the thalamus, striatum, and cerebellum. Within the local cortical network (within a few tens of millimeters), cortical neurons synchronously depolarize and hyperpolarize during the slow oscillations.

3.3 The slow oscillation is a traveling wave

Studies monitoring the distribution of selected slow oscillation phases reveal that the timing of the negative peak exhibits a continuous shift that can be traced spatially throughout the cortex. On average, the maximum delay across the cortex, calculated by determining the difference between the negative peak of the initial slow-wave trace to the negative peak of the terminal trace is about 120 msec. Additionally, slow oscillations originate more frequently in anterior regions and propagate posteriorly. Streamline maps that condense the spatio-temporal dynamics of the slow oscillation display an origin density that coincides with the positioning of anterior electrodes, while the average delay map assumes a predominant fronto-occipital direction of propagation. Importantly, the pattern of origin and propagation of slow oscillations is reproducible across time and across subjects.

Taken together, these studies show that post-learning sleep occurs across the cortex leading to a slight increase in firing in a small set of neurons whose activity is causally linked to neuroplasticity learning, with an activity synchronized and much greater decrease in firing of a larger set of neurons not involved in neuroplastic modulation, consistent with the renormalization hypothesis.

3.4 The cyclical nature of sleep

A third implication of the current sleep hypotheses is the cyclical character of renormalization events, which are dictated by the ongoing twin needs of neuroplastic learning during wakeful periods and of replenishment during sleep. The temporal organization of these cycles follows nature's light/dark rhythms, where the overall balance in total synaptic strength is maintained across the circadian 24-hour sleep/wake cycle with its temporally regulated, reoccurrence of similar events.

3.5 Circadian rhythms

Based on the presence of this pattern, the fields of circadian biology and sleep–wake regulation have been closely linked for decades, with studies exploring how the circadian clock regulates daily rhythms in sleep and wakefulness, and in turn, how arousal levels in animals affect their circadian clocks. Despite their close relationship, the two, nonetheless, are physiologically independent. Collectively, they may be understood as a homeostatic process – the plastic, organizational events of wakefulness and the dissociative, restorative events of sleep – and the circadian clock-like mechanisms that temporally govern the distribution of wakefulness and sleep periods in synchrony with the external environment [27]. While the two systems have been shown to share elements of their mechanisms, in other aspects the two display many distinct features, evident in their anatomical, molecular, and electrophysiological details.

The preeminent circadian clock in mammals is located in the suprachiasmatic nucleus (SCN), immediately above the optic chiasm and juxtaposed with the third ventricle. Lesions of the SCN eliminate daily rhythms such as the sleep–wake rhythm [28]. The SCN circadian oscillator consists of a transcriptional-translational negative feedback loop (TTFL), involving a group of clock genes that includes Period (Per) 1 and 2; Cryptochrome (Cry) 1 and 2, Brain and muscle Arnt-like-1 (Bmal1), and Clock. While the SCN clock phase is modulated by many inputs the primary environmental synchronizer is light stimulation via the retina, which is then relayed to the SCN. Circadian mechanisms regulating sleep include SCN efferents to the subparaventricular zone, which sends excitatory projections to the medial preoptic and dorsomedial hypothalamus, the latter of which sends additional excitatory projections to LH orexin neurons and to the LC [27]. SCN neuronal activity is higher in the day, with initial output from the SCN excitatory in diurnal animals. Distinct from the circadian signals emanating from the SCN, there are also distributed circadian influences on sleep. For example, the circadian clock gene Bmal1 regulates the rhythmic production of histamine in wake-promoting tuberomammillary neurons. Selective Bmal1 deletion in these neurons, renders them arrhythmic. Another circadian clock gene, Reverbα, regulates circadian dopamine production in the VTA.

Unlike the SCN circadian clock, the sleep–wake system is distributed across many brain regions, including the brainstem, midbrain, hypothalamus, thalamus, and cortex. Moreover, sleep is composed of a complex mixture of different brain states, having their unique electrical recording features. Broadly these include slow-wave sleep, i.e., non rapid eye movement sleep (NREM), characterized by high amplitude, low-frequency brain waves, and rapid eye movement sleep (REMS), defined by low amplitude, higher frequency EEG activity, with mixtures of these occurring during transitional phases [29]. The nature of the homeostatic "process" is less clear than that of circadian rhythms, and likely encompasses multiple factors. Examples of postulated molecules include extracellular adenosine, which has been shown to increase during the wake in parallel with higher metabolic activity and to decrease during sleep as metabolism wanes [30]; prostaglandin D2, which also accumulates during wake, activates DP1 receptors and increases extracellular adenosine levels; and cytokines such as interleukin (IL)-1β and tumor necrosis factor (TNF)α. Central to the concept of "process" is that sleep serves a restorative function that allows the brain to consolidate synaptic changes generated by previous events, replenish energy stores, and eliminate accumulated metabolic byproducts [12]. Although the circadian and sleep–wake systems are quite distinct, it is noteworthy that they share many cellular processes. Accumulating evidence supports both systems utilizing extracellular processes that overlap the synaptic mechanisms associated with learning, memory, and drug addiction, including changes in enzymatic activity, morphological changes associated with the extracellular matrix (ECM) and ECM-associated proteins, and astrocyte-associated processes [31].

4. The arousal system and the modulation of global up and down states

4.1 The arousal system

The universality of sleep implies the need for precise mechanisms that enable renormalization as well as the transitioning therefrom to wakeful periods of interactive learning. Insight into these mechanisms has emerged from studies of trauma lesions in humans, pharmacological experimentation in mammalian species, and in situ preparations. Together, they have revealed a critical dependence of sleep-like states on the modulation of arousal systems, with the inhibition of neurotransmitters like GABA leading to sleep and their stimulation to wakefulness. While these have to date been the primary mechanisms identified for transitioning between sleep stages, other work has also revealed physiological mechanisms that act directly to induce sleep.

Characteristic of the trauma observations is the case of a 39-year-old man [32] who suffered head trauma resulting from a car collision. Immediately after the head trauma incident, the patient complained of excessive sleepiness and sudden muscle weakness of all four extremities. At three months after onset, his Epworth Sleepiness Scale score was 19, which has a normal range of 10. Diffusion tensor imaging data of the *ascending reticular activating system* (ARAS) showed that the tract volume of the right ventral lower ARAS was substantially decreased compared with control subjects indicating neural trauma to the structure at the site between the pontine RF and the hypothalamus, thus revealing the involvement of the ARAS in sleep modulation.

Consistent with such trauma observations, data from many laboratories has demonstrated that GABAergic transmission in the PnO promotes wakefulness [33]. Inhibiting GABAergic transmission in the PnO by microinjection of the GABA synthesis inhibitor (3-MPA), for instance, decreases anesthesia induction time with isoflurane and/or propofol. Elevating GABA levels with the uptake inhibitor (NPA) into the PnO reverses this effect. On the other hand, modulation of GABA levels in the PnO does not alter the time to recovery of anesthesia. These data provide support for the conclusion that modulation of arousal is a primary mechanism for transitioning between sleep stages, while the lack of effect on the emergence from anesthesia implicates a more complex process for this aspect of arousal than GABA modulation alone.

In addition to GABA the peptides hypocretin-1 and -2, termed orexin A and B, also modulate sleep stage transitioning via the arousal system [34]. Similar to the case of GABA receptors, receptors for the hypocretins are site-specific and widely dispersed. Cell bodies of hypocretin-producing neurons have been localized to the dorsolateral hypothalamus but send projections to all the major brain regions that regulate arousal. Hypocretin-1 delivered to rat dorsal raphé nucleus increases serotonin release in the dorsal raphé and to the pontine nucleus increases acetylcholine and GABA levels, suggesting that the peptide may broadly activate neurotransmitter release as a function of brain location.

Few studies have revealed a direct induction of sleep via neurotransmitter upregulation. Of these, REM sleep was induced in rats using vasoactive intestinal polypeptide (VIP). A closely related peptide, the pituitary adenylyl cyclase-activating polypeptide (PACAP), was even more effective [35]. The IC_{50} for PACAP was 2.4 and 3.2 nM, for example, as compared with VIP $IC_{50} > 1$ mM, suggesting the peptide has a highly specific and effective role in the induction of REM sleep regulation. In an interesting observation, injection of PACAP into the PnO generated REM sleep lasting 11 consecutive days.

4.2 Targeting the arousal system

Due to an improving understanding of the regulatory mechanisms for sleep transitions, pharmacotherapy has chiefly emphasized the evolution of drugs targeting receptors for neurotransmitters of the arousal system. These are briefly discussed with regard to the selectivity of their effects and the specificity of their interactions with sleep phases.

4.2.1 GABA, regional influences, and NREM sleep

Because of their powerful inhibitory effects, $GABA_A$ receptors have been the targets of most sedative/hypnotic and general anesthetic drugs. $GABA_A$ receptors exist as multiple subtypes and these subtypes are differentially located throughout the brain. The differences in clinical effects caused by various benzodiazepine (e.g., diazepam) and non-benzodiazepine (e.g., eszopiclone) sedative/hypnotics are attributed to the relative selectivity for different $GABA_A$ receptor subtypes. For example, administering the benzodiazepine site agonists zolpidem, diazepam, and eszopiclone directly into the PnO caused drug-specific changes in cortical electroencephalographic activity and increased acetylcholine release in the PnO [11]. Systemic administration of eszopiclone to awake rats significantly decreased acetylcholine release in the PnO and increased electroencephalographic power in the delta frequency. These data suggest that different classes of clinically used sedative-hypnotics can exert their arousal-modulating effects by actions at different GABAA receptors in the PnO.

On the other hand, the development of sedative/hypnotic pharmaceuticals has largely been empiric, leading to the present consecutive evolution from the benzodiazepines, the initial drugs of choice, which were limited by their addiction potential. The empiric approach has produced clinically useful drugs but has not generated drugs with a comprehensive range of desirable properties. Nonetheless, the identification and characterization of receptor subtypes, the regional distribution of their siting within the brain, a growing ability to modify and simulate sleep architecture, improved knowledge of the physiological features that distinguish sleep phases, and technological advances in drug delivery hold promise for more selective therapeutic intervention. As mentioned, for example, systemic administration of GABA mimetic drugs is known to promote sleep, sedation, or general anesthesia. In brain regions containing neurons that promote wakefulness, GABAergic inhibition has been shown to cause an increase in sleep. These brain regions include the dorsal raphé nucleus and the tuberomamillary nucleus of the posterior hypothalamus, for example. Yet, direct administration into the pontine reticular formation of drugs that increase GABAergic transmission increases wakefulness and inhibits sleep.

4.2.2 Acetylcholine and REM sleep

Although acetylcholine plays a primary role in generating the brain-activated states of wakefulness and REM sleep, cholinergic drugs are not part of the standard pharmacological armamentarium of sleep disorders medicine. Nonetheless, understanding the mechanisms by which cholinergic neurotransmission generates and maintains REM sleep is crucial, because of its selective influence on this phase of sleep architecture as well as its interaction with other transmitter systems that are targets of sleep pharmacotherapy [11].

Much of the research on the regulation of sleep by acetylcholine has focused on transmission mediated by muscarinic cholinergic receptors. Of the five subtypes (M_1–M_5) of muscarinic receptors that have been identified, the M2 subtype plays a key role in the generation of REM sleep. Cholinergic signaling originating from the laterodorsal tegmental and pedunculopontine tegmental nuclei (LDT/PPT) and the basal forebrain promotes the cortically activated states of wakefulness and REM sleep. The distinction between sleep phases has been shown to be due to the presence of two cortical populations of neurons that induce either wakefulness and REM sleep (referred to as Wake-On/REM-On) or wakefulness alone (Wake-On/REM-Off).

In vivo data obtained from normal rats demonstrate that the sedative/hypnotics zolpidem, diazepam, and eszopiclone differentially alter acetylcholine release in the pontine nucleus, increase EEG delta power, and decrease acetylcholine release in rat pontine reticular formation. Intravenous administration of eszopiclone, for instance, prevents the REM phase of sleep, increases EEG delta power, and decreases acetylcholine release in rat pontine reticular formation.

5. Sleep dysfunction and dysfunctional system states

5.1 Global dysfunction

5.1.1 Psychiatric diseases

Psychiatric diseases are often conceptualized as broadly linked to global brain states, and so subject to the influences of global sleep disturbances. Several examples indicate that sleep disturbances comprise etiological factors resulting in psychiatric dysfunctions [36].

In adolescents at high-risk (UHR) for psychosis, for example, the study of the relationships between sleep disturbances and psychosis symptoms, the volume of an integral sleep structure (thalamus), and associations between thalamic abnormalities and sleep impairment in UHR youth an increased latency to sleep onset and greater sleep disturbances/disrupted continuity compared to normal youth, over and above concurrent mood symptoms. Among UHR youth, increased sleep dysfunction was associated with greater negative symptom severity. Compared to HC adolescents, UHR participants displayed decreased bilateral thalamus volume, which appeared to be correlated with increased sleep dysfunction.

Slow waves and sleep spindles are the two main oscillations occurring during NREM sleep. While slow oscillations are primarily generated and modulated by the cortex, sleep spindles are initiated by the thalamic reticular nucleus (TRN) and regulated by thalamo-reticular and thalamo-cortical circuits. Monitoring these distinct electrical signatures in 18 medicated schizophrenics revealed reduced sleep spindles compared to healthy and depressed subjects during the first NREM episode. Whole night hd-EEG recordings from a larger patient cohort revealed whole-night deficits in spindle power (12–16 Hz) and in slow (12–14 Hz) and fast (14–16 Hz) spindle amplitude, duration, number, and integrated spindle activity (ISA) in prefrontal, centroparietal and temporal regions. By contrast, no slow wave deficits were found in schizophrenics. These results indicate that spindle deficits can be reliably established in schizophrenics and are stable across the night, suggesting deficits in TRN and thalamo- reticular circuits *unrelated* to antipsychotic medications.

It is widely known that children and adolescents with autism spectrum disorders (ASD) suffer from sleep disorders. These include increased bedtime resistance, insomnia, awakening, parasomnia, sleep-breathing disorders, and waking difficulties. Frequently, the sleep disorder appears first, suggesting that sleep is a causal factor in ASD development [7]. Abnormal behaviors from future ASD patients have been recognized in the newborn period. These display sleep disorders preceding the onset of ASD.

5.2 Impaired regulation of sensorial input

5.2.1 Learning impairments due to disturbances that affect slow oscillations in NREM sleep

A key postulate of current sleep models is the restorative effect of sleep on learning in brain areas that have experienced heavy neuroplastic changes during wakeful periods. This postulate was tested in experiments that focally perturbed deep sleep in the motor cortex and investigated the consequences on behavioral and neurophysiological markers of neuroplasticity related to motor practice. The restoration in the ability to learn was markedly attenuated in these experiments when slow waves were selectively perturbed in the motor cortex. This demonstrated that deep sleep – specifically its electrical signature – was needed to maintain the ability to learn efficiently after recovery from sleep and that disturbances of sleep like insomnia would therefore be likely to impede learning.

5.2.2 Cyclical irregularities affect autonomic balance and addiction

Disorders in sleep rhythms are increasingly commonly encountered in pediatric and adolescent populations. Characteristic clinical features include familial advanced sleep phase syndrome (ASPS) and delayed sleep phase syndrome (DSPS), non-24-h sleep–wake syndrome (non-24), and morningness-eveningness recognition. Accompanying these rhythm irregularities are severe fatigue and gastrointestinal discomfort [2] that appear to be due to autonomic imbalances.

Cyclical irregularities appear to also impact dopaminergic brain regions that are substantially associated with addiction. In investigations of the midbrain ventral tegmental area (VTA) neural activity recordings exhibited a strong vigilance state with increased activity during wakefulness and rapid eye movement sleep relative to non-rapid eye movement sleep. Six hours of sleep deprivation induced a significant depression of neuronal activity in both areas. Surprisingly, these alterations lasted for up to 48 hours and persisted even after the normalization of cortical EEG waves. These results show that sleep disturbances significantly affect neuronal activity in midbrain DA structures and so are likely to reflect the frequently observed relationship between sleep alterations and dysfunction of the DA circuitry observed in addiction [37].

6. Conclusion

The clear implication from the current theoretical picture of sleep is that its influence is fundamental to many neuronal systems. As such its properties are key to understanding how sleep broadly affects brain function and systemic well-being. To date, however, the ability to assess this influence has lacked experimental tools having sufficient precision to characterize these systems. This circumstance is gradually in the process of resolution as the ongoing expansion in the pharmacopeia of sleep medications continues.

While the data describing these medications offer a sobering reminder of the complexity that must be logically integrated if we are to derive a coherent model of the processes regulating sleep, it is simultaneously a cogent argument that the manipulation of these mechanisms now has the potential for refined control. Indeed, today's pharmacopeia presents a spectrum of drugs tailored to various sleep features.

The focus on the use of these medications is likely to demonstrate the cross-cutting relevance of sleep for the practice of medicine in numerous neurological issues. The pressing clinical problem of sleep disorders medicine will thus continue to stimulate advances in understanding not merely the neurochemical regulation of sleep but also the health of the brain's broader neurological functioning.

Author details

Denis Larrivee[1,2]

1 Mind and Brain Institute, University of Navarra Medical School, Spain

2 Loyola University Chicago, USA

*Address all correspondence to: sallar1@aol.com

References

[1] Noda A, Yasuma F, Okada T, et al. Circadian rhythm of autonomic activity in patients with obstructive sleep apnea syndrome. Clinical Cardiology. 1998;**21**:271-276

[2] Tomoda A, Miike T, Yonamine K, et al. Disturbed circadian core body temperature rhythm and sleep disturbance in school refusal children and adolescents. Biological Psychiatry. 1997;**41**:810-813

[3] Toyoura M, Miike T, Tajima S, et al. Inadequate sleep as a contributor to impaired glucose tolerance: A cross-sectional study in children, adolescents, and young adults with circadian rhythm sleep-wake disorder. Pediatric Diabetes. 2020 Jun;**21**(4):557-564

[4] Lunsford-Avery JR, Mittal VA. Sleep dysfunction prior to the onset of schizophrenia: A review and neurodevelopmental diathesis–stress conceptualization Clinical Psychology: Science and Practice. 2013;**20**:291-320

[5] Massimini M, Huber R, Ferrarelli F, Hill S, Tononi G. The sleep slow oscillation as a traveling wave. The Journal of Neuroscience. 2004;**24**(31):6862-6870

[6] Ismail FY, Fatemi A, Johnston MV. Cerebral plasticity: Windows of opportunity in the developing brain. European Journal of Paediatric Neurology. 2017;**21**:23-48

[7] Peiper NC, Ridenour TA, Fishbein DH. Characterizing psychiatric symptoms and neurocognitive functioning among substance-naïve early adolescents: Associations with sleep problems. Early Intervention in Psychiatry. 2020;**14**:439-449

[8] Brower KJ, Perron BE. Sleep disturbance as a universal risk factor for relapse in addictions to psychoactive substances. Medical Hypotheses. 2010;**74**:928-933

[9] Feld GB, Born BJ. Neurochemical mechanisms for memory processing during sleep: Basic findings in humans and neuropsychiatric implications. Neuropsychopharmacology. 2020;**45**: 31-44. DOI: 10.1038/s41386-019-0490-9

[10] Vadnie CA, McClung CA. Circadian rhythm disturbances in mood disorders: Insights into the role of the suprachiasmatic nucleus. Hindawi Neuroplasticity. 2017;**11**(5):28. DOI: 10.1155/2017/1504507

[11] Watson CJ, Baghdoyan HA, Lydic R. Neuropharmacology of sleep and wakefulness: 2012 update. Sleep Medicine Clinics. 2012;**7**(3):469-486. DOI: 10.1016/j.jsmc.2012.06.010

[12] Tononi G, Cirelli C. Sleep and synaptic down-selection. The European Journal of Neuroscience. 2020;**51**:413-421

[13] Aton SJ, Broussard C, Dumoulin M, Seibt J, Watson A, Coleman T, et al. Visual experience and subsequent sleep induce sequential plastic changes in putative inhibitory and excitatory cortical neurons. Proceedings of the National Academy of Sciences of the United States of America. 2013;**110**:3101-3106

[14] Goel N, Rao H, Durmer JS, Dinges DF. Neurocognitive consequences of sleep deprivation. Seminars in Neurology. 2009;**29**: 320-339

[15] Kirchhoff M, Parr T, Palacios E, Friston K, Kiverstein J. The Markov blankets of life: autonomy, Active inference and the free energy principle. Journal of the Royal Society Interface. 2018;**15**:20170792. DOI: 10.1098/rsif.2017.0792

[16] Friston K, Sengupta B, Auletta G. Cognitive dynamics: From attractors to active inference. Proceedings of the IEEE. 2014;**102**(4):427-446

[17] Bedau M. The nature of life. In: Boden M, editor. The Philosophy of Artificial Life. Vol. c1966. Oxford: Oxford University Press; 1996. pp. 332-360

[18] Tononi G, Cirelli C. Some considerations on sleep and neural plasticity. Archives Italiennes de Biologie. 2001;**139**:221-241

[19] Cirelli C, Tononi G. Effects of sleep and waking on the synaptic ultrastructure. Philosophical Transactions of the Royal Society B. 2020;**375**:20190235

[20] Bjorness TE, Kulkarni A, Rybalchenko V, Suzuki A, Bridges C, Harrington AJ, et al. An essential role for MEF2C in the cortical response to loss of sleep in mice. eLife. 2020;**9**:1

[21] Flavell SW, Cowan CW, Kim TK, Greer PL, Lin Y, Paradis S, et al. Activity-dependent regulation of MEF2 transcription factors suppresses excitatory synapse number. Science. 2006;**31**:11008-11012

[22] Lante F, Toledo-Salas JC, Ondrejcak T, Rowan MJ, Ulrich D. Removal of synaptic Ca(2)+−permeable AMPA receptors during sleep. The Journal of Neuroscience. 2011;**31**:3953-3961

[23] Gulati T, Guo L, Ramanathan DS, Bodepudi A, Ganguly K. Neural reactivations during sleep determine network credit assignment. Nature Neuroscience. 2017;**20**:1277-1284. DOI: doi. org/10.1038/nn.4601

[24] Norimoto H, Makino K, Gao M, Shikano Y, Okamoto K, Ishikawa T, et al. Hippocampal ripples down-regulate synapses. Science. 2018;**359**:1524-1527

[25] Girardeau G, Benchenane K, Wiener SI, Buzsaki G, Zugaro MB. Selective suppression of hippocampal ripples impairs spatial memory. Nature Neuroscience. 2009;**12**:1222-1223. DOI: doi. org/10.1038/nn.2384

[26] Steriade M, Timofeev I, Grenier F. Natural waking and sleep states: A view from inside neocortical neurons. Journal of Neurophysiology. 2001;**85**:1969-1985. DOI: doi.org/10.1152/jn.2001.85.5.1969

[27] Borbely AA, Daan S, Wirz-Justice A, Deboer T. The two-process model of sleep regulation: A reappraisal. Journal of Sleep Research. 2016;**25**:131-143

[28] Moore RY. Organization of the mammalian circadian system. Ciba Foundation Symposium. 1995; **1995**(183):88-106

[29] Scammell TE, Arrigoni E, Lipton JO. Neural circuitry of wakefulness and sleep. Neuron. 2017;**93**:747-765

[30] Holst SC, Landolt HP. Sleep homeostasis, metabolism, and adenosine. Current Sleep Medicine Reports. 2015;**1**:27-37

[31] Panja D, Bramham CR. BDNF mechanisms in late LTP formation: A synthesis and breakdown. Neuropharmacology. 2014;**2014**(76): 664-676

[32] Jang SH, Seo WS, Hyeok KG. Post-traumatic narcolepsy and injury of the ascending reticular activating system. Sleep Medicine. 2016;**17**:124-125

[33] Vanini G, Watson CJ, Soto-Calderon H, Lydic R, Baghdoyan HA. GABA levels in cat pontine reticular formation (PRF) and pedunculopontine tegmental nucleus (PPT) vary with arousal state. In: Neuroscience Meeting Planner 458.15. Atlanta, GA Soc Neurosci. 2006

[34] Wang C, Wang Q, Ji B, Pan Y, Xu C, Cheng B, et al. The orexin receptor system: Molecular mechanism and

therapeutic potential for neurological diseases. Frontiers in Molecular Neuroscience. 2018;**11**:220. DOI: 10.3389/fnmol.2018.00220

[35] Ahnaou A, Basille M, Gonzalez B, Vaudry H, Hamon M, Adrienand J, et al. Long-term enhancement of REM sleep by the pituitary adenylyl cyclase-activating polypeptide (PACAP) in the pontine reticular formation of the rat. The European Journal of Neuroscience. 1999;**11**:4051-4058

[36] Lunsford-Avery JR, Orr JM, Gupta T, Pelletier-Baldelli A, Dean DJ, Smith Watts AK, et al. Sleep dysfunction and thalamic abnormalities in adolescents at ultra high-risk for psychosis. Schizophrenia Research. 2013;**151**(151):148-153

[37] Fifel K, Johanna H, Meijer JH, Deboer T. Circadian and homeostatic modulation of multi-unit activity in midbrain dopaminergic structures. Scientific Reports. 2018;**8**:7765. DOI: 10.1038/s41598-018-25770-5

Chapter 2

Neurophysiology of Basic Molecules Affecting Sleep and Wakefulness Mechanisms, Fundamentals of Sleep Pharmacology

Murat Kayabekir

Abstract

As part of the biological rhythm, the human brain has a healthy functioning with the ability to differentiate between day and night hours in any given day (sleep rhythm, life rhythm). From the control of hormone levels to muscle tonus, from the regulation of respiratory rate to the content of our thoughts, sleep has an impact on all bodily and cognitive functions. It is not surprising to see such effects of sleep on the body as it leads to significant changes in the electrical activity of the brain in general. Electrical signal changes in the brain (sleep-wakefulness rhythm) are regulated by neurohormonal molecules and their receptors in the body. Neurotransmitters that control sleep and wakefulness can be listed as "Glutamate, Acetylcholine, Histamine, Norepinephrine and GABA". Main hormones are: Melatonin, Corticotropin Releasing Hormone (CRH), cortisol, prolactin, Growth Hormone (GH), Insulin like Growth Factor (IGF-1, Somatomedin-C), Follicle Stimulating Hormone (FSH) and Luteinizing Hormone (LH), progesterone, estrogen, testosterone, catecholamines, leptin and neuropeptide Y". The effects of pharmacological agents on sleep and wakefulness cycles are materialized through the following molecules and their receptors: Hypnotics (GABA A agonists, benzodiazepines, gabapentin, tiagabine), sedative antidepressants (tricyclic antidepressants, trazadone, mitrazapine), antihistamines, medications used for the treatment of sleeplessness (melatonin and melatonin analogues), amphetamine (most commonly used stimulant), secretion of monoamines (dopamine), non-amphetamine stimulants used in the treatment of hypersomnia and narcolepsy (modafinil, bupropion, selegiline, caffeine) and other substances (alcohol, nicotine, anesthetics). To the extent we can conceptualize the physiological mechanisms of these basic molecules listed above and the regions they affect, we can appreciate the effects of these substances on sleep physiology and sleep disorders.

Keywords: sleep-wakefulness rhythm, major neurohormones, neurophysiological effects of sleep-wakefulness molecules, basic sleep pharmacology

1. Introduction

A healthy interaction between wakefulness and sleep periods and a balance specific to the organism is necessary for the proper functioning of human physiology and specifically that of the central nervous system (CNS) to be maintained. Sleep is a physiological need, it is a behavior during which the response of the brain to environmental stimuli is reversibly diminished. The absence or diminishment of this need negatively impacts the interactions in the neuronal networks and pathways responsible for the wakefulness of the brain. Electrical activity changes that appear in the brain during NREM and REM periods with the help of neurohumoral factors gives way to different physiological mechanisms in the body. Motor networks are integrated during REM, and non-motor ones during NREM. Thus, diseases that affect bodily organs and systems as well as medications can change NREM and REM activities thereby changing the motor and sensory functions of the brain. We can easily claim that many basic and clinical neurophysiological incidents taking place when we are awake are in fact realized through physiological processes and pathophysiological mechanisms occurring during sleep. Anxiety disorders, depression and schizophrenia where neurotransmitter-receptor relationships are hindered, as well as motor and non-motor degenerative diseases (Amyotrophic Lateral Sclerosis, Parkinson's disease) present with sleep disturbances and REM behavior changes years ahead of clinical symptoms. Sleep is as important a piece of life as wakefulness. As we continue to understand sleep, many of the causes of basic and clinical processes from pediatric age to geriatric years will be further demystified.

2. Neurophysiology of basic molecules affecting sleep and wakefulness mechanisms, fundamentals of sleep pharmacology

2.1 The relationship between behavior, limbic system and autonomous nervous system

When we talk about brain, we think about cortex; when cortex is mentioned, we focus on somatosensory (senses) and somatomotor (movement) cortex activities; when we hear about hypothalamus, we then consider hypothalamopituitary hormones and feedback mechanisms. Yet, humans are not limited to biological functions. Behavior is what defines a human being. Physiological and social characteristics associated with behaviors and even habits can influence the diseases individuals develop and the treatment approaches that are used. The emergence of behavior is managed by the limbic system which in itself means limit. Hypothalamus is at the center of the limbic system; rather than primarily focusing on biological-feedback interactions, it plays a key role in the integration and control of behavior [1–3]. The most important element of sleep and wakefulness cycle is our behavior model. Sleep is the most basic physiological need and the most important electrical activity of the brain influencing wakefulness behaviors (thirst, hunger, satiety, emotional state, mood, social motivation, love, compassion, argument, fear, attention, concentration, learning, memory and many other cognitive, motor, sensory and autonomous functions) [2–5]. Deep brain has hypothalamus at its center and it orchestrates affective sensations (like/dislike, satisfaction/revulsion, reward/punishment) together with surrounding limbic structures. As the main center of integration, hypothalamus uses parasympathetic and sympathetic fibers of the autonomous nervous system generating vegetative, emotional and motivational mechanisms. Amygdala is the main limbic structure for emotions: (1) it stimulates sympathetic activity, especially previously learned fear-related behavior. (2) Can be voluntary, when the cerebral cortex decides to recall frightful experiences it acts through amygdala. (3) Some people can regulate some autonomic activities by gaining extraordinary control over their emotions. (4) It is sensitive to sleep deprivation that is why you get cranky when you have not slept enough. Reticular formation of brain stem, regulation of pupil size, respiration, heart, blood pressure, swallowing etc. Sleep/wakefulness cycle is a complex blend of all these physiological and behavioral processes. There are two distinct stages during sleep: a stage where there are no rapid eye movements NREM (Non Rapid Eye Movement) and one where there are rapid eye movements REM (Rapid Eye Movement). These stages are separated from one another and from wakefulness with hard limits [4–8].

2.2 Neuroanatomy of sleep and wakefulness behavior

There are two main regions (mesopontine reticular activating system **(RAS) and hypothalamus**; these two central regions modulate the intralaminar thalamus and neurons found in the basal forebrain) and a circadian pacemaker (**Suprachiasmatic Nucleus (SCN)**) with a central role that regulate the sleep and wakefulness cycle: **RAS** stimulates the cortex by ventral and dorsal tracts. Ventral tract stimulates the frontal parts of the brain through hypothalamus and subthalamus, dorsal tract stimulates it through the nucleus groups in the thalamus. During wakefulness, transmission of sensory information from thalamus is permitted through RAS control managed by thalamus. During sleep, the activity of RAS stops and the transmission of sensory information through thalamus is blocked and the stimulation of cortex is prevented. **Anatomic structures responsible for the hypothalamic control of sleep and wakefulness:** for wakefulness, stimuli originating from rostral pons and caudal midbrain regions reach paramedian midbrain in diencephalon and here, the signals divide into two paths aiming to reach thalamus and hypothalamus. Main structures projecting to thalamus are PedinculoPontine Tegmental (PPT) and LateroDorsal Tegmental (LDT) nuclei that are of cholinergic nature. The structure that initiates sleep is thought to be the ventrolateral preoptic nucleus (VLPO) located on the anterior part of the hypothalamus. VLPO suppresses the activities of brain stem, pons and locus coeruleus (LC), dorsal raphe nucleus (RN), laterodorsal tegmental pedinculopontine tegmental nucleus via GABA and galanine neurotransmitters. **Suprachiasmatic Nucleus (SCN)** is known as the light sensitive circadian pacemaker. During daytime, light stimulus is transmitted from retina to hypothalamus through neural pathways and it results in the secretion of melatonin from the pineal gland. It is an anatomical structure that has a central role in maintaining the day-night rhythm [1, 9–11]. It is multisynaptic and sympathetic nervous system contributes to this.

2.3 Physiology of neurotransmitters for sleep and wakefulness

2.3.1 Basic neurotransmitters for sleep and wakefulness cycle and a neurohormone

Dopamine: It is synthesized from L-Dopa with aromatic L-amino acid decarboxylase enzyme (cofactor pyridoxine). Dopamine receptors: D1 receptor; is found on nigrostriatal pathway specifically on nucleus caudatus, it plays a role on the initiation of locomotor system movements. D2 receptor; is found prominently in striatum and mesolimbic pathways, it plays a role in motor effects associated with extrapyramidal system. D3 receptor; is mostly found in the limbic system, it plays an important role in emotional and cognitive processes. D4 receptor; is increased in number in schizophrenia. D5 receptor; is important for the dopamine/acetylcholine balance in the basal ganglia and in maintaining a normal somatomotor and striated muscle tone. Parkinson and Huntington chorea are prototypic diseases for decreased and increased dopaminergic activity, respectively. Dopamine decreases the secretions of prolactin and TRH [12–14].

Serotonin (5-hydroxytriptamine, 5-HT): L-Tryptophan is converted into 5-hydroxytryptamine (5-HT) with tryptophan hydroxylase (5-hydroxytryptophane) and amino acid decarboxylase enzymes. Most of the serotonergic pathways are found within the Raphe system (2 pathways) in the brain. **(1) Ascending pathway:** Regulation of feeding behavior (decreases the appetite together with histamine and nicotine), continuation of normal behavioral patterns, regulation of-NREM-REM sleep cycle, hormonal regulation (increases ACTH and prolactin secretions, decreases GnRH secretion), depression, anxiety and migraine pathogenesis. **(2) Descending pathway**: Acts as a modulator in the transmission of pain sensation to the central level. Serotonin receptors: 5HT1-A: Shows an anxiolytic effect. 5HT1-B: It is a presynaptic inhibitor. 5HT1-D: Closes the AV shunts in the brain, plays a role in migraine pathogenesis. 5HT2: Has excitatory effects on behavior. 5HT2-C: Specifically found in choroid plexus where atypical antipsychotic clozapine exerts its effects. 5HT3: Stimulates the respiratory center and is found in the autonomous nervous system. 5HT4: Primarily found in the myenteric plexus within the gastrointestinal system [12–14].

Adenosine: It is a nucleoside naturally found in all bodily cells. It forms molecules like adenosine triphosphate (ATP) and adenosine diphosphate (ADP) to transmit energy inside the cells; at the same time, it is one of the chemical messengers (xanthine) or neurotransmitters in the brain. It is a substance that is produced either directly or as a result of ATP hydrolysis. It is broken down by adenosine deaminase. It has 2 known receptors: P1 (A1–4) and (A1 and A2 receptors are blocked by methyl xanthines) P2X-2Y. It has depressant effects on the CNS. As an inhibitor transmitter in the brain, it shows an incremental increase specifically in RAS throughout the wakefulness period; when it reaches its highest level, adenosine inhibition takes place, sleep starts and adenosine concentration gradually decreases during sleep. Caffeine blocks the depressant effects of adenosine on the brain, decreases adenosine inhibition and provides for the continuation of wakefulness while carbamazepine (adenosine agonist, antiepileptic) helps to continue adenosine inhibition [15–17].

Melatonin (A neurohormone that identifies daytime and nighttime): It plays an important role in identifying the circadian rhythm. It is synthesized from 5-HT in the pineal gland by acetyltransferase and methyltransferase enzymes. Melatonin receptors are mostly found in SCN. The physiological actions of melatonin are mediated by two G-protein coupled membrane receptors, which belong to the family of the quinone reductases. Melatonin receptors: MT1; is primarily found in the human skin. It is associated with the aging process and Alzheimer's disease. MT1 and MT2 receptors are expressed in the SCN and they have distinct functional roles in sleep regulation. Activation of the MT1 receptor suppresses neuronal firing rates in the SCN, while MT2 mainly acts by inducing circadian rhythm phase shifts. MT2; has anxiolytic, antidepressant and hypnotic effects and is related to pain pathophysiology. MT3; is related to quinone reductase enzyme and it plays a role in the prevention of stress as well as detoxification [18–20].

2.3.2 Neurotransmitters in charge of sleep and wakefulness

"Glutamate, Acetylcholine, Histamine, Norepinephrine and GABA".

Glutamate: It is the main excitatory neurotransmitter in the brain and medulla spinalis. Its inactive form is glutamine. It plays a primary role in the generation of excitatory postsynaptic potentials and long-term potentiation in the brain and these are the most important mechanisms in learning and memory formation. Its most important receptors are: NMDA (N-methyl-D-aspartate; it is a Na^{+}-K^{+}-Ca^{++} channel type receptor, its selective antagonist is phencyclidine and its endogenous blocker is Mg^{++}), AMPA (alpha-amino-3-hydroxy-5 methyl-4- isoxazole propionic acid), Kainate (kainic asid) receptors (KARs) [12–13].

Acetylcholine: It has muscarinic and nicotinic receptors in the CNS. Nearly 80% of the cholinergic pathways in the brain originate from Meynert's nucleus basalis. Nicotinic receptors are mainly found in Renshaw cells that inhibit alpha motor neurons in medulla spinalis. In addition to learning and memory functions, they also play a role in the balanced functioning of the extrapyramidal system. A parallelism has been shown between the degeneration of this pathway and the occurrence of Alzheimer's disease and Huntington chorea [12–14].

Histamine: Ventral posterior hypothalamus and tuberomamillary nucleus (TMN) receiving histaminergic projections have the highest concentrations of histaminergic neurons in the brain. H1 receptors are found in glial cells and H3 receptors are in basal ganglia. Serotonin-like effects of histamine are: (1) to decrease the appetite and (2) to increase the secretion of ACTH and prolactin [13, 14].

Norepinephrine: In the CNS, catecholaminergic neurons are most abundant in locus coeruleus. The highest concentrations of norepinephrine are found in hypothalamus, nucleus amygdala and the dentate gyrus of hippocampus. Medullar reticular formation harbors the highest levels of epinephrine. It has Beta 1 and 2 activator receptors which are widespread in the CNS. Alpha 1 causes vigilance (behavioral activations). Alpha 2 acts as an autoreceptor at presynaptic level and is inhibitory in nature (sedation). The activation of this system in the CNS leads to panic reaction presenting with alertness, fear and a state of alarm. Furthermore, it causes anxiety and tremor. However, the decrease in the efficacy of this system leads to depression. Catecholamines also increase the secretions of GnRH and ACTH [12–14].

Gamma-Aminobutyric Acid (GABA): It is the main inhibitory mediator of the brain. GABA is synthesized from glutamic acid by glutamic acid decarboxylase enzyme (activated by valproic acid). The main route of its inactivation in the synaptic space is re-uptake and it is broken into succinic acid semialdehyde by the GABA transaminase enzyme (inhibited by vigabatrin). It has two receptors of inhibitory character: (1) GABA-A receptor is a chlorine channel. When it is activated, due to the influx of the Cl ions, intracellular negativity increases (hyperpolarization). This receptor has 5 subunits (2 alpha, 2 beta, 1 gamma): The agonist for the beta subunit is muscimol, its antagonist is bicuculline; alpha subunit is a benzodiazepine receptor. Barbiturate is a Cl channel agonist, while picrotoxin and pentylenetetrazole are antagonists. It has binding regions for ethanol and ivermectin. (2) GABA-B receptor is not of ion channel character. It is not affected by benzodiazepines or barbiturates. It is activated by baclofen and antagonized by faclofen and saclofen [14–16].

2.3.3 Mechanism of action of neurotransmitters on sleep and wakefulness neurons

Reticular activating system stimulates the cortex by utilizing glutamate while ponto-mesencephalic tegmental neurons do this by using acetylcholine. Neurons at locus coeruleus predominantly utilize norepinephrine, they extend from the brain stem to the cerebral cortex encompassing the forebrain; by activating the stimulation of the cortex, and they contribute to maintaining wakefulness. **Cholinergic neuronal network** leads to wakefulness in two types of cortexes:

1. It projects to laterodorsal tegmental and pedinculopontine tegmental nuclei, midline and intralaminar thalamic nuclei and to a lesser degree to lateral hypothalamus and basal forebrain.

2. Cholinergic neuron group starts from the basal forebrain with a widespread projection to cortex. This pontomesencephalic neuron group is a part of the ascending reticular activating system; they play a part in the activation during wakefulness and are actively involved in paradoxical sleep. Glutamate is another excitatory neurotransmitter acting as the primary neurotransmitter of the ascending reticular activating system. **Glutamate** is found at very high concentrations at the brainstem reticular formation. It plays an active role in the wakeful brain and is secreted from the cortical cells during wakefulness. During deep sleep, slow wave sleep (SWS) "burst discharges" appear as a result of the activation of special glutamate receptors. Histamine plays an important role in wakefulness as well. **Histamine containing neurons** are found in tuberomammillary nuclei and posterior hypothalamus. **Noradrenergic neurons** (locus coeruleus), have diffuse projections in the brain extending to the cortex. Histaminergic neurons are associated with cortical activation during wakefulness while they are shut down during REM sleep. Sleep requires a shift from sympathetic regulation to parasympathetic regulation. Parasympathetic centers of significance are located in "solitary tract nucleus neurons, anterior hypothalamus and preoptic fields". When increasing **adenosine** concentrations in RAS reach their highest levels, **serotonergic raphe neurons** facilitate the beginning of sleep while **GABA-ergic neurons** inhibit the activating system. These GABA-ergic neurons are selectively activated during SWS. As a result of this inhibition, brain stem, hypothalamus and nasal forebrain are suppressed and disfacilitation (inhibition) and hyperpolarization of thalamocortical system takes place. Thereby, from the wakeful state where we see rapid, tonic discharges on EEG, the system shifts into sleep state where we start recording sleep spindles and slow wave activity. Initiation and continuation of SWS is made possible by lengthening and strengthening the inhibition of the activating system with GABA-ergic system. Metabolic rate of adenosine dictates sensitivity to sleep deprivation while directly influencing the quality and duration of SWS [6, 9, 20–25].

2.3.4 The physiology of the circadian system and melatonin in the regulation of circadian rhythm

In Latin, circa means pertaining to and dian means day; circadian is a word used to explain the daily physiological rhythms of an organism, mainly the sleep and wakefulness.

The anatomy of the circadian rhythm: The regions in charge of the circadian rhythm in mammals are the right and the left suprachiasmatic nuclei (SCN) located in the anterior hypothalamus. SCN is divided into ventrolateral and dorsomedial sections on the basis of biochemical structure, peptide phenotypes and afferent-efferent pathways. SCN is affected by environmental changes such as light and time of nutrition. SCN also has functional regions that regulate circadian rhythm outputs associated with neural activity. Light is perceived by retinal photoreceptors (cones, rods, retinal ganglion cells containing melanopsin). The action potentials that are generated here lead to the secretion of glutamate and pituitary adenylate cyclase activating polypeptide via retinohypothalamic pathways. Information about light intensity and temporal stimulus is directly transmitted to SNC while it is indirectly transferred to the lateral geniculate region in the thalamus. SCN receives significant inputs from serotonergic median raphe nucleus and intergeniculate region containing neuropeptide Y and GABA (These regions are not essential for circadian rhythm; however, they transfer information about light sensitive phase changes and stimulants other than light to the circadian rhythm center). The effects of light on SCN activity and circadian phase changes are completely opposite of those of neuropeptide Y and serotonin. As the center of circadian rhythm, SCN contributes to the regulation of behavioral, physiological and genetic rhythms. The most important aspect is its relationship with hypothalamus; (1) Main neuronal pathway regulating sleep-wakefulness rhythm SCN – neighboring supraventricular region, SCN-dorsomedial hypothalamic region (2) SCN-sends both direct and indirect fibers to paraventricular hypothalamic nucleus regulating corticosteroid secretion and melatonin synthesis. The regulation of the circadian rhythm improves the adaptation of the organism to life; towards the end of a night's sleep, body temperature, plasma cortisol levels and sympathetic autonomous activity all increase. When sleep time approaches, body temperature decreases and melatonin secretion starts. In mammals, circadian rhythm center at SCN regulates the phases and timings of all cyclical behavioral functions together with sleep-wakefulness cycle. Identifying the neuronal pathways and neurotransmitters playing a role in this regulation is crucial for developing pharmacological and strategical approaches for chronobiological sleep disorders [25–27]. **Melatonin in the regulation of sleep and circadian rhythm:** Melatonin is the neuroendocrine modulator of day-night rhythm with receptors densely located at the suprachiasmatic nucleus (SCN). The endogenous circadian rhythm of melatonin secretion is directly proportional to the endogenous rhythm of sleep tendency. Secretion of melatonin from the pineal gland is controlled by SCN. This pathway is multisynaptic and has contributions from the sympathetic nervous system. When administered to the body from outside melatonin helps initiate sleep; as it leads to phase shifts, it has therapeutic effects in insomnia and regulation of sleep-wakefulness phases. The biological clock can be regarded as an insurance preventing sleep phase shifts caused by homeostatic changes. When human beings intend to change the timing of sleep-wakefulness rhythms at their own will (most common causes are travels to regions with time differences and working with shifts), insomnia ensues. **Sleep regulation, Homeostasis, Sleep homeostasis and Sleep-wakefulness rhythm:** Three main processes play a role in sleep regulation: (1) Homeostatic process which tells us the relationship between the last sleep and wakefulness periods. In sleep deprived organisms the duration and depth of sleep increases as a compensatory mechanism. (2) Circadian process; in other words the biological clock. (3) Ultradian process which defines the duration of REM—NREM sleep cycles and the interactions between them. Sleep wakefulness rhythm is identified by circadian and homeostatic processes. Homeostasis is the preservation of required internal environment conditions (extracellular fluid) for maintaining the vitality of the organism. Sleep homeostasis is the equivalent of sleep-wakefulness balance in sleep regulation. This balance is maintained by homeostatic mechanisms and deviations from the normal are either normalized or brought closer to normal. Circadian process can be regarded as an internal clock that lasts 24 hours. Homeostatic process is related to the time spent awake before sleeping. Therefore, there are three important features of a medication to be used in the treatment of insomnia caused by circadian clock changes: (1) Hypnotic effect: the ability to initiate or to maintain sleep when homeostatic effect is inadequate to do so. (2) Chronohypnotic effect: the ability to inhibit the time of waking-up normally regulated by the circadian center. (3) Chronobiotic effect: concerning the regulation of the circadian rhythm, the ability to initiate phase shifts and to do so during desired hours. **Melatonin** is a hormone that harbors all these three features.

Secretion of melatonin from the pineal gland is controlled by SCN. Furthermore, it is multisynaptic and has contributions from the CNS. If there is light exposure during night hours, melatonin levels decrease immediately. Melatonin levels are influenced by certain medications: Beta blockers used for the prophylaxis of hypertension, cardiac arrhythmias and headaches block the sympathetic activity both at the heart and at the pineal gland. On the other hand, antidepressant drug fluvoxamine prevents the degradation of melatonin and increases its plasma concentrations. Administration of 0.3–80 mg oral melatonin during daytime when endogenous melatonin levels are low, will decrease sleep latency and have a sleep inducing effect. Melatonin effect is related to body posture; it increases when lying down and decreases when standing up. Neurotransmitter imbalance is present in SCN of essential hypertension patients and there is a decrease in the secretion of melatonin in coronary artery disease that follows. In patients with uncontrolled hypertension, taking 2.5 mg of melatonin 1 hour before sleep is shown to increase the total duration and the efficacy of sleep. **EEG pattern of sleep regulation:** Sleep regulation is mainly identified by sleep homeostasis: in sleep deprivation, the length of sleep increases and it gets deeper as a compensatory mechanism. Because sleep needs are identified by the homeostatic and circadian processes. As the time spent awake before sleeping increases, slow waves in sleep EEG increase and sleep spindles decrease. Neurophysiologically, thalamocortical neurons have a moderate level hyperpolarization during the superficial stages of NREM sleep (N1 and N2) and high level of polarization during deep stages (N3) of NREM. During superficial NREM sleep, there are more frequent thalamocortical discharges and EEG equivalent of these are sleep spindles. Theta activity in awake EEG shows the homeostatic process. As the period spent awake gets longer, theta activity increases and SWS (delta) activity increases to the same extent. Despite the fact that their mechanisms of action are different, similar to benzodiazepines the use of melatonin suppresses low frequency EEG activity [27–29].

2.4 The effects of sleep and circadian rhythm on hormones

Circadian rhythmicity and sleep-wakefulness homeostasis includes; (1) the modulation of hypothalamic hormones, peptides and molecules, (2) the metabolic pathways influenced by peripheral hormones and (3) autonomous nervous system control of endocrine organs. In the regulation of temporal organization of hormone secretion, processes associated with the electrical signal changes during the sleep stages of brain (NREM-REM) are as effective as circadian rhythm and homeostatic processes. These processes effect different hormonal axes (somatotropic, corticotropic and gonadal axes) and metabolic pathways at different levels. For example thyroid stimulating hormone (TSH) levels might change both with sleep and circadian rhythm while cortisol levels only change with circadian rhythm. Growth hormone (GH) and prolactin (PRL) can be at a certain level during daytime- wakefulness but they increase while sleeping. Glucose and insulin have been shown to be effected by both sleep and the circadian rhythm increasing while being awake at night and while being asleep during daytime. Circadian oscillations can be generated in many peripheral organs under autonomous nervous system control including adipocytes and pancreas beta cells that generate endocrine signals. These "local" oscillators seem to be under the control of central electrical batteries found in suprachiasmatic nuclei either directly through neural and endocrine signals or indirectly via sleep-wakefulness cycle and behavioral rhythms like nutrition. Endocrine secretion of these peripheral oscillators during wakefulness and sleep and their possible participation in the temporal organization of metabolic function are still open to research [30–32].

2.4.1 Somatotropic axis and sleep

Growth Hormone (GH): Pituitary secretion of GH is stimulated by hypothalamic GH secreting hormone (GHRH) and is inhibited by somatostatin. Acylated form of ghrelin that is predominantly produced in the stomach binds to growth hormone secreting (GHS) receptors and endogenously stimulates GH secretion. GH is a respiratory stimulant. Animal studies have shown that the infusions of GHRH and ghrelin result in SWS, while GH infusion leads to REM sleep. There is a consistent relationship between the presence of Delta waves on EEG and high concentrations of GH and maximum GH secretion takes place minutes after the start of SWS. Pharmacological agents used in narcolepsy like gamma hydroxyl butyrate (GHB) and ritanserin that stimulate SWS cause an increase in GH. Sleep-initiated GH secretion is regulated by GHRH stimulation that primarily takes place during somatotropin inhibition where somatotropic activity decreases. Secretion of GH during early sleep is suppressed by the administration of a GHRH antagonist [15]. SWS decreases with age and there are also medical conditions that result in sleep fragmentation which all decrease GH secretion. Sleep deprivation effects GH secretion through deteriorations in both the circadian rhythm and sleep-wakefulness homeostasis. **Insulin like Growth Factor (IGF-1) (Somatomedin C):** It is a hormone primarily synthesized in the liver by being stimulated with GH. It mediates the anabolizing effects of GH in the muscle tissue. In men it decreased after 21 years of age while there is a rapid decline in women after menopause. It is a respiratory stimulant like GH and leads to increases in SWS. **Somatostatin:** Inhibits the GHRH stimulation of GH secretion. It has a suppressive effect on the respiratory center and is thought to play a role in sudden infant death syndrome [33–35].

2.4.2 Corticotropic axis and sleep

The activity of the corticotropic axis is related to stress reaction and behavioral activation. Corticotropic axis activity can be measured peripherally by plasma levels of pituitary adrenocorticotropic hormone (ACTH) and adrenal hormone cortisol that is directly controlled by ACTH stimulation. Plasma levels of these hormones are highest during early hours of morning, they decrease throughout the day reaching lowest limit during late night hours and early stages of sleep period. Therefore, sleep is normally initiates when corticotropic activity is slow. Reactivation of ACTH and cortisol secretion happens suddenly a couple of hours ahead of waking up. **Corticotropin releasing hormone (CRH):** It regulates GnRH secretion and stimulates adrenocorticotropic hormone secretion (ACTH) from the pituitary gland. It binds to CRH receptors that are abundant in the brain and stimulates breathing. In instances of stress it acts as a part of hypothalamo pituitary adrenal axis and increases plasma cortisol levels. **Cortisol:** Physiologically low levels of cortisol at the beginning of sleep is correlated with SWS and cortisol secretion mostly starts during superficial stages of sleep. When there is sleep deprivation, cortisol levels act in parallel to circadian rhythm increasing and decreasing at the same time; however, as there is a change in the time sleep starts and ends, cortisol levels are somewhat higher during nighttime (where it should be lower), and somewhat lower during the day (where it should be higher) (thus the amplitude of cortisol rhythm decreases). In elderly individuals with fragmented sleep and decreased SWS, worsened memory and insulin resistance that is observed is related to the increased cortisol levels at night. Waking up during fragmented sleep results in increases in cortisone levels (as concerns cortisol increase and sleep fragmentation, it is not clear which one is the cause and which is the result). Cushing patients were shown to have bad sleep quality, decreases in REM latency, increases in first REM intensity and decreases in deep sleep. Addison patients also had decreases in deep sleep. Therefore, we can conclude that for deep sleep to happen, the organism needs cortisol rhythm within normal limits [36–38].

2.4.3 Thyrotropic axis and sleep

Thyroid Stimulating Hormone (TSH)-Triiodothyronine (T3)-Thyroxine (T4): It is stable throughout the day and increases during the early hours of the evening reaching its maximum level at the beginning of sleep. Before waking up in the morning, it returns to its stable levels that continue through the day. TSH secretion is influenced by the circadian rhythm and by sleep. Sleep had an inhibitory effect on TSH. This effect disappears during sleep deprivation, nocturnal TSH levels increase together with increases in T3 and T4. Thyroid hormones are respiratory stimulants. In hypothyroidism, there is a tendency for hypoventilation and obstructive apnea syndrome. There is sleepiness during daytime and decreases in SWS. In hyperthyroidism, there is increased movement during sleep, decreased REM duration and insomnia due to increased metabolic rate [39, 40].

2.4.4 Prolactin (PRL) and sleep

PRL levels begin to increase shortly after the start of sleep and make a night peak at the middle of sleep. The possible primary mechanism underlying this peak is decreased dopaminergic inhibition of PRL during sleep. Thyrotropin releasing hormone (TRH), vasoactive intestinal peptide (VIP), oxytocin, estrogen and angiotensin II increase PRL secretion while dopamine, GABA and acute hypoxia inhibits it. The primary effect of PRL during sleep is to stimulate REM sleep. Rapid PRL increase at the beginning of sleep is thought to be related to SWS. In prolactinoma and lactating mothers SWS increases due to increased PRL secretion. Fragmented sleep decreases PRL secretion (Mechanism: Waking up in the morning and wakefulness that fragment sleep are related to a rapid inhibition of PRL secretion) [41, 42].

2.4.5 Gonadal axis and sleep

The relationship between 24-hour-gonadotropin secretion rhythms and gonadal steroid levels changes based on the stage of maturity and is sex-related during young adulthood [42].

Gonadotropins: Before puberty, luteinizing hormone (LH) and follicle stimulating hormone (FSH), is secreted in a pulsatile fashion both in boys and girls. Increased amplitude of gonadotropin secretion during sleep is a distinctive characteristic of adolescence. In adolescent girls, estradiol levels are higher during the day than the night; in adolescent boys high levels of testosterone during nighttime coincide with increases in gonadotropins. Both sleep and circadian rhythm contribute to the increases in gonadotropin pulsations during the night in adolescents. As they transition into adulthood, the effect of circadian rhythm either decreases or disappears completely. In sleep deprivation, LH increases, FSH does not change. Adult 24-hour plasma LH levels are regulated by the menstrual cycle in women, in men it changes according to NREM-REM cycles. In young men, REM sleep deprivation weakens night increases of testosterone in particular. In elderly men, there is a decrease in LH secretion during sleep while it increases in elderly women; however this is not in relation with the circadian rhythm. **Progesterone:** It increases during pregnancy and during the luteal phase of menstrual cycle. As it is a respiratory stimulant, there are low carbon dioxide levels and hyperventilation during these periods. When progesterone decreases during the postmenopausal period, nocturnal desaturation, hypopnea and apneas are seen more frequently. In individuals administered with estrogen and progesterone during postmenopausal period, sleep breathing disorders were less common. **Estrogen:** In young women, it is at its lowest level during menstruation and at its highest during the midluteal phase (estradiol). It is in the form of estrone during postmenopause. Estradiol increases the effects of progesterone on respiration by increasing the number of progesterone receptors. **Testosterone:** Despite the low amplitude of nighttime increase in gonadotropin secretion, there is a significant diurnal rhythm for testosterone levels in the circulation. Testosterone is at its lowest levels during the late hours of the night; after sleep starts, there is a strong increase and it reaches its maximum levels during the early hours of the morning [51, 52]. Therefore, the strong circadian rhythm of plasma testosterone can be partially controlled by factors other than LH. Nighttime increase of testosterone is temporarily related to the delay of first REM episode. There are studies showing that sleep breathing problems are due to decreased levels of testosterone during nighttime as well as those showing that respiratory stimulation is decreased by the negative effect on progesterone [43–46].

2.4.6 Catecholaminergic axis and sleep

With initiation of sleep, noradrenaline and adrenaline levels decrease as the case with cortisol reaching their minimum levels within an hour. Noradrenaline plays a role in respiratory control while adrenaline is a bronchodilator. Nocturnal catecholamine levels are increased in patients with obstructive apnea syndrome.

2.5 Physiological mechanisms of basic molecules that cause sleep related metabolic changes

2.5.1 Molecules mediating nutrition and sleep regulation

Sleep plays an important role in energy balance. Hypocretins and orexins are hypothalamic stimulant neuropeptides with strong wakefulness promoting effects, they also stimulate feeding; their definition created the molecular basis for delineating the interactions between nutrition and sleep regulation.

Orexin: Orexin containing neurons in lateral hypothalamus directly lead to locus coeruleus and other brainstem and hypothalamic stimulation areas; here they interact with leptin sensitive neuronal network which plays a role in balancing food intake and energy consumption. Orexin containing neurons are active when awake and inactive when asleep. Orexin activity is inhibited by leptin which is a satiety hormone and stimulated by ghrelin, an appetite stimulating hormone. **Leptin:** Leptin is a hormone secreted by adipocytes, it provides information to the regulating centers at hypothalamus about energy status. Nighttime increases of leptin is thought to suppress hunger during night fasting. When administered systemically, it causes increases in SWS and decreases in REM. As it inhibits Neuropeptide Y (suppresses respiration) secretion, it stimulates corticotropin releasing hormone-CRH (stimulates respiration) secretion. Research trials have shown that it stimulated respiration and that CPAP (continuous positive air pressure) treatment decreased leptin receptor sensitivity. Long term total sleep deprivation decreases leptin levels. **Ghrelin:** It plays a role in regulating energy balance and stimulating appetite. Ghrelin levels increase sharply before each fixed meal time and make a nadir 1–2 hours after eating. Although hunger continues, ghrelin levels do not continue to increase throughout sleep and decreases during later hours of sleep instead. When at high levels during sleep, it is a strong endogenous stimulant of GH secretion [43, 47–49]. **Neuropeptide Y (NPY):** NPY is widely distributed in hypothalamus, amygdala, locus coeruleus and cerebral cortex. At least six NPY receptor subtypes have been defined. NPY plays a role in food intake, hormonal secretion, circadian rhythms, stress reaction, anxiety and sleep functions. In animals, depending on the site of injection, NPY was found to have sleep promoting effects as well as wakefulness effects. In humans, NPY is thought to have hypnotic characteristics and act as a physiological antagonist of CRH. NPY participates in the timing of sleep onset in humans and can thus play a role in the integration of sleep regulation, food intake and metabolism [43, 50].

2.5.2 Autonomic nervous system co-transmitters (neuropeptides)

Nuclei located in hypothalamus (posterior and lateral regions contain sympathetic nuclei, anterior regions have parasympathetic ones) control the autonomic nervous system. Together with hypothalamus and limbic structures, sympathetic and parasympathetic portions of the autonomic nervous system regulate vegetative sensory and motivational behaviors. Norepinephrine (noradrenaline) is the main transmitter for the sympathetic system (catecholaminergic system), and Neuropeptide Y acts as a cotransmitter. In vascular beds, adrenergic endings secrete NPY together with noradrenaline. By itself, NPY has a vasoconstrictor effect. Acetylcholine (Ach) is the main transmitter of the parasympathetic system (cholinergic system) and VIP (vasoactive intestinal peptide) functions as the cotransmitter of this system. In the salivary and perspiratory glands, in the genital system and adrenal medulla cholinergic endings secrete VIP together with ACh. VIP exerts partial vasodilator and strong bronchodilator effects [7, 12–14].

2.5.3 Melanin-concentrating hormone (MCH)

MCH, is a 19 amino acid long cyclic neuropeptide acting as a neurotransmitter. Neurons containing MCH are primarily found in lateral hypothalamus and incerto-hypothalamic regions and they have widespread projections within the brain. In humans, biological functions of this neuropeptide are realized via two metabotropic receptors, namely MCHR1 and MCHR2, whereas rodents only have MCHR1. **General functions in the organism**: **(1)** Feeding behavior and energy conservation; high concentrations of MCH, might lead to increased eating and is associated with increases in body mass. On the contrary, decreases in existing levels of MCH can lead to decreased eating. Increased MCH levels in olfactory regions have been associated with the consumption of oily foods with high calorie content. Good tasting food items promote MCH encouraging higher consumption of them. Sugar, specifically glucose seems to be supporting the role of MCH in sleep and energy conservation. Supporting energy conservation in this manner has been associated with high body mass even when the diet is under control. **(2)** Having MCH at certain locations only during lactation seems to help promote maternal behavior. **(3)** Reproduction: MCH has been assumed to act as a modulator in Luteinizing Hormone (LH) secretion by having a direct effect on the pituitary gland or by indirectly influencing gonadotropin releasing hormone (GNRH) in the hypothalamus. Estrogen seems to be required for MCH to influence reproduction. **(4)** Skin pigmentation: MCHR1 has been found in human melanocytes and certain melanoma cells. In these cells, it has an antagonistic relationship with α-MSH and it decreases melanin production. **Specific regulation of sleep behavior:** As concerns the sleep cycle, MCH and orexin have an antagonistic relationship with one another, orexin is nearly totally active during wakefulness periods and MCH is more active. MCHergic neurons are more active during sleep, specifically during REM sleep; although they increase SWS as well, they mainly increase the duration of REM sleep. MCH knockout mice have shorter REM sleep especially under negative energy balance circumstances. Systemically administered MCHR1 antagonists decrease sleep. While MCH promotes sleep, there are limited number of studies associating MCH with narcolepsy. Narcolepsy has long been described as a disorder of REM sleep mechanism. An individual with narcolepsy starts sleeping with REM sleep. Narcolepsy presents with the loss of hypothalamic cells that contain hypocretin and orexin. A research study has demonstrated that individuals having narcolepsy had diminished orexin neurons that would promote wakefulness and that the number of MCH neurons was not different than those of an average individual who does not have narcolepsy. MCH has been associated with depression and anxiety. MCHR1 antagonists were shown to act as antidepressants [1]. Chemokines and cytokines generally appear as a result of inflammation or infection and can then damage MCH neurons thereby possibly causing anorexia in an individual. MCH has been identified both in melanoma and squamous cell carcinoma cell lines [43, 51–54].

2.6 Overview (a general look at sleep related neuropharmacology)

The system and molecules that are in charge of regulating sleep-wakefulness modulate general homeostatic mechanisms as well as orchestrating highly cognitive activities like attention, learning and memory. We need to develop a general perspective for pharmacologic substances influencing these activities.

2.6.1 Alcohol

Ethyl alcohol; blocks glutamate NMDA receptors and is an indirect agonist of GABA receptors. Cerebral granular cells increase GABAergic transmission in cerebellar cortex and hippocampus. Alcohol is neurotoxic at high doses; it can specifically hinder cholinergic input that advances to the cortex through basal forebrain neurons. It can lead to a significant deterioration in motor performance and can result in sleep deprivation. There might be behavioral problems stemming from sleep deficiency as well as memory problems in alcoholics because of apparent effects of alcohol on hippocampus. Individuals having undiagnosed schizophrenia, anxiety disorders and depression might try to benefit from sedative and anxiolytic effects of alcohol by overconsumption. In these individuals, blood circulation to the frontal region deteriorates and their decision making capacity is impaired [14, 15].

2.6.2 Anesthetics, sedatives and hypnotics

Main mechanisms of effect for sleep inducing pharmacological agents are still being delineated. The primary site of action of most anesthetics may be the sleep–wake control system. In anesthesia, considering that arousal and alertness represent a continuum of levels from mania to coma, with physiological and behavioral concomitants, the monitoring of EEG, along with behavioral and autonomic signs, should be used routinely to assess level of anesthesia. **Most anesthetics**, including barbiturates, etomide, propofol, neuroactive steroids, and volatile anesthetics, act on GABAa receptors among other receptors. Sedation and natural sleep occur greatly as a result of enhanced GABAergic transmission, which in turn affects the release of a number of excitatory transmitters such as acetylcholine, excitatory amino acids, and histamine. Actions may take place specifically in such regions as the RAS, TMN, and basal forebrain (all of which have local circuit GABAergic neurons and receive GABAergic input from VLPO, as described earlier), thereby regulating the level of arousal. The benzodiazepines act by binding to a site that modulates GABA receptors, especially GABAa receptors. These agents produce sedative, hypnotic, anxiolytic, and anticonvulsant activities. They act generally by amplifying GABAergic transmission, such that short-acting agents have been used to promote sleep in insomnia patients, although more recently, effective non-benzodiazepine hypnotics have been developed. These agents also act to facilitate GABAa receptor function (e.g., zolpidem and zaleplon). Insomnia is a very common symptom, especially in the elderly, and has a number of causes, including physical, social, and psychiatric. **Antidepressants with sedative effects** (**tricyclic** antidepressants, trazadone, nefazadone and mitrazapine) exert their effects on emotional state via 5-HT norepinephrine (NE) receptors, their sedative effects are seen through H1, 5-HT2, alpha1 receptor antagonisms. **Drugs used in insomnia treatment** (melatonin and melatonin analogues) exert their effects via MT1 and MT2 receptors. **Other hypnotic substances acting through GABA** (Valerian preparations, Gabapentin, Tiagabine), **Sedative antipsychotics** (Olanzapine, quetiapine; they are 5HT-2A antagonists), **Gamma hydroxybutyrate** (its mechanism of effect is not fully understood, it is considered to modulate dopamine activity; it is recommended in narcolepsy for cataplexy treatment) [14, 15, 55, 56].

2.6.3 Antihistamines

Histaminergic projections at tuberomamillary nucleus are active during waking up. The pathology of this region leads to hypersomnia. Histaminergic inputs coming from TMN to RAS suppress SWS, but they do not have an effect on REM. RAS, basal forebrain, lateral hypothalamus and cortex have high levels of histamine receptors. Antihistamine (histamine receptor blockers) effects on these regions cause dizziness, sleepiness and cognitive dysfunction. In children first and second generation antihistamines can cause poisoning and coma; however, newer (third generation) pediatric formulations (e.g. fexofenadine, loratadine, cetirizine) seem to be safer [57].

2.6.4 Caffeine

The popularity of caffeine is due to its stimulant characteristics. It blocks adenosine receptors in RAS, decreases the inhibitor effect of adenosine; thus, free adenosine levels in the brain are increased resulting in a stimulant activity in the CNS. Caffeine appears to block adenosine A1 and A2a receptors, producing a psychomotor stimulant effect. Because of the high levels of A2a receptors in the striatum, the potential use of caffeine for the treatment of Parkinson's disease has been advanced. Since adenosine A2a receptor blockade appears to protect dopaminergic neurons from toxic agents, a neuroprotective role has been proposed for caffeine in the treatment of Parkinson's disease. Caffeine intake has also been associated with a decreased risk of Alzheimer's disease, again presumably acting as a neuroprotective agent [12].

2.6.5 Nicotine

It is an alkaloid found in abundance in tobacco and eggplants. It is metabolized in the liver and its main metabolite is cotinine. With smoking low dosed of nicotine exerts its effects on sympathetic (tachycardia, high blood pressure) and parasympathetic (tonus in the digestive system, increases in peristaltic movements and acid secretion) effects. (Thromboxane A2 increase, lipolysis, psychomotor stimulation, decreases appetite, analgesic effect, increases the secretion of ADH, ACTH, cortisol and insulin, decreases secretion of LH and PRL). Causes psychological and physical addiction. Inhaled nicotine in cigarette smoke is known to permeate the lungs where more than 80% of the available nicotine is absorbed into the bloodstream. After absorption into the blood, nicotine readily crosses the blood– brain barrier and appears to be rapidly partitioned into brain tissue. Concentrations of nicotine in the brain have been reported to be 5–7 times higher than blood concentrations. Smokers assert that, in addition to its positive effects on concentration and attention, the primary positive effect of smoking is that it calms and relaxes. Recent findings suggest that one of the sites of action of nicotine may be in the RAS, specifically, on PPN neurons. Nicotine, at least initially, has an inhibitory effect on cholinergic RAS neurons, which could produce the calming effect reported upon inhalation of cigarette smoke. The majority of cigarettes are consumed by the mentally ill, especially those with disorders involving hypervigilance or hyperarousal, such as schizophrenia, anxiety disorders, and depression. That is, smoking may be a form of self-medication, presumably because of its calming effects. This effect (inhibition of cholinergic RAS neurons) appears to differ from the role of smoking in reducing the incidence of Parkinson's disease, which appears to be manifested as a neuroprotective action on dopaminergic neurons by nicotine. Cerebral vasodilation is seen immediately after smoking, but chronic smokers show global reductions in cerebral blood flow. Considering that hypofrontality is present in schizophrenia, anxiety disorders, and depression, the initial beneficial, calming effects of nicotine may be followed by deleterious consequences on cortical blood flow. Such an effect may drive craving for the next cigarette, creating a vicious cycle of continuous self-administration [12, 58, 59].

2.6.6 Stimulants

The most commonly used stimulant, amphetamine, induces release of monoamines, especially dopamine, but also blocks their reuptake and may have neurotoxic effects on nigral neurons and, more recently, is suspected of inducing the degenerations of certain striatal neurons. Unfortunately, this agent is abused for recreational purposes and continues to be prescribed for the treatment of attention deficit disorder (ADD). Fortunately, methylphenidate does not appear to have such neurotoxic effects, although its use has decreased.

Non-amphetamine stimulants: Modafinil- has been specifically produced for the treatment of narcolepsy. Modafinil is a newer stimulant that does not appear to act through dopaminergic mechanisms, like amphetamine. Modafinil does seems to affect structures involved in the regulation of sleep– wake states and to affect a number of transmitter systems, including noradrenergic, histaminergic, and orexinergic, as well as excitatory amino acid and serotonin release. In addition, it may block GABAa receptors [60–62].

2.6.7 Schizophrenia, anxiety disorder and depression

Hypofrontality, hypervigilance and sleep irregularities are common symptoms for these disorders. Regions in relation with RAS (cholinergic PPN, noradrenergic LC and serotonergic RN) that we tried to tackle so far, their neurotransmitters and pharmacological agents that are effective on their receptors are used for the treatment of these symptoms. The serotonergic RN is known to inhibit the PPN and LC, with the cholinergic PPN exciting the LC and the noradrenergic LC inhibiting, via alpha-2 adrenergic receptors, the PPN. The PPN sends excitatory cholinergic projections to the substantia nigra (SN), which, in turn, sends dopaminergic projections to the striatum. The treatment of depression previously included tricyclic antidepressants such as amitryptiline, imipramine, and clomipramine, agents that mainly blocked reuptake of noradrenaline and serotonin, and blocked histamine and acetylcholine release, thus accounting for increased sleepiness. The selective serotonin reuptake inhibitors (SSRIs) more selectively affect the RAS by increasing the inhibition. It is not clear if the etiology of depression is related to disinhibition of the PPN and LC by a decrement in serotonergic tone, although this would seem a likely origin for the sleep–wake symptomatology of depression. The treatment of anxiety disorder is involved the use of benzodiazepine amplification of GABAergic inhibition. In addition, the use of the alpha-2 noradrenergic receptor agonist clonidine produces anxiolytic effects, probably by inhibiting autoreceptors in the LC and postsynaptic receptors in the PPN, thus downregulating vigilance. Because of the peripheral cardiovascular effects of clonidine, alpha-2 adrenergic receptor agonists without such actions would be more desirable. One study provided strong evidence for the use of the alpha-2 adrenergic receptor agonist dexmedetomidine as an anxiolytic for the treatment of anxiety disorders like posttraumatic stress disorder, panic attacks, and general anxiety disorder [32]. The etiology of anxiety disorder has been proposed to include downregulation or degeneration of LC outputs (possibly induced by stress hormones), which would act to release, or disinhibit, PPN neurons at site.

The etiology of schizophrenia has been suggested to include increased PPN output, accounting for marked hypervigilance and hallucinations. Excessive PPN output would overactivate the SN and, in turn, increase striatal release of dopamine that is, complying with the dopamine theory of schziophrenia. SWS are reduced in schizophrenics. Consistent with this assumption, lower SWA has been more often reported in institutionalized patients with profound cognitive impairment as well as in schizophrenia patients with prominent negative symptoms. The treatment of schizophrenia previously involved the use of the dopaminergic receptor blocker haloperidol, which induced tardive dyskinesia, among other serious side effects. Newer antipsychotics such as risperidone and quetiapine appear to block dopaminergic, noradrenergic, and serotonergic receptors. More striking antipsychotic effects were provided by the use of clozapine, which was designed as a muscarinic cholinergic blocker for the treatment of Parkinson's disease [14, 63–65].

2.6.8 Motor and non-motor degenerative diseases (amyotrophic lateral sclerosis, Parkinson's disease)

ALS is an incurable neurodegenerative disorder of upper and lower motor neurons, which is characterized by degeneration of the corticospinal tracts, resulting in loss of motor neurons in the brain, brainstem and anterior horn cells of the spinal cord. Loss of motor neurons in the brainstem and spinal cord causes weakness of the pharyngeal, laryngeal, intercostal and diaphragmatic muscles. During non-REM sleep, muscle tone is decreased and during REM sleep muscle tone is almost completely lost. Automatic ventilation during sleep is almost completely dependent on the diaphragm (particularly in REM sleep) therefore diaphragmatic dysfunction (such as that seen in ALS) can predispose to hypoventilation and nocturnal hypoxemia. Parkinson Disease [PD] is the second most common neurodegenerative disorder after Alzheimer's disease. PD occurs as a result of chronic, progressive decrease in dopamine levels of the substantia nigra, secondary to loss of dopaminergic neurons in the pars compacta and the occurrence of Lewy bodies in the cytoplasm of remaining neurons. It is primarily diagnosed clinically and patients may present with the characteristic motor deficits, which include the resting tremor, bradykinesia, rigidity and postural instability. However, most will have both motor and nonmotor symptoms. The nonmotor symptoms cause disturbances, which affect sleep, mood, cognition, sensation and autonomic function. Among the nonmotor symptoms in PD, sleep disorders are second in frequency only to neuropsychiatric disorder [16, 65–68].

2.6.9 Analytical functions of molecules affecting sleep in neurophysiology and physiopathology

Particular attention to hormonal conditions is warranted. After all, the first sign of puberty is pulsatile hormone (LH) release during sleep. For example, narcolepsy is tightly linked with certain human leukocyte antigen (HLA) haplotypes, suggesting that it is an autoimmune disorder. Kleine– Levin syndrome, discussed earlier, is linked to similar haplotypes, which suggests an autoimmune etiology. Interestingly, in most cases of narcolepsy, Kleine– Levin syndrome, as well as schizophrenia, panic attacks, obsessive– compulsive disorder, and other disorders, the age of onset is soon after puberty. Along other lines, in about 20% of schizophrenic patients, the mother had an influenza attack during the second trimester, while narcoleptics are born predominantly during the late winter– early spring, that is, after influenza season. It has been suggested that developmental dysregulation, either pre- or perinatally (initial insult), becomes pathologically manifest after exposure to puberty and its hormonal onslaught. These considerations point to complex interactions between development, environment, and hormonal status, all of which seem to affect sleep– wake regulation in as yet unknown ways. These findings suggest that the effects of hormones, either prescribed or taken as dietary supplements, or abused, need to be more closely studied and considered in the design of therapeutic interventions [69, 70].

Brain energy requirements are extraordinarily high; any modification in glucose utilization by the brain may profoundly affect glucose tolerance. Cerebral glucose utilization is lower during SWS than during either REM sleep or wake. Using PET scans, a strong correlation was evidenced between slow-wave activity, an index of the intensity of SWS, and regional blood flow in the prefrontal brain. Furthermore, experimental studies, involving continuous enteral nutrition or intravenous glucose infusion while allowing for normal nocturnal sleep, have shown that glucose tolerance is minimal during the first half of the sleep period, i.e. when SWS is the dominant sleep stage. These findings confirm the existence of a robust link between SWS and glucose tolerance. Both reduction in total sleep duration with slow-wave sleep (SWS) largely preserved and alterations of sleep quality (especially marked reduction of SWS) with preservation of total sleep duration areassociated with insulin resistance without compensatory increase in insulin secretion, resulting in impaired glucose tolerance and increased risk of type 2 diabetes. When performed under rigorously controlled conditions of energy intake and physical activity, sleep restriction is also associated with a decrease in circulating levels of leptin (an anorexigenic hormone) and an increase in circulating levels of ghrelin (an orexigenic hormone), hunger and appetite. Furthermore, sleep restriction is also associated with a stimulation of brain regions sensitive to food stimuli, indicating that sleep loss may lead to obesity through the selection of high-calorie food. There is also evidence that sleep restriction could provide a permissive environment for the activation of genes that promote obesity. Indeed, the heritability of body mass index is increased in short sleepers. Thus, chronic sleep curtailment, which is on the rise in modern society, including in children, is likely to contribute to the current epidemics of type 2 diabetes and obesity [71–73].

Chronic sleep loss is increasingly common in industrialized societies, affecting about 45% of adults. Sleep deprivation induces behavioral, hormonal, and neurochemical alterations. The stress inherent in sleep deprivation causes changes in the concentration of hormones such as cortisol as well as in prolactin and estradiol, which are known to influence dopaminergic transmission.

Studies have suggested that dopamine (DA) is responsible for the behavioral changes observed after sleep deprivation. Specifically, REM sleep deprivation has been shown to be related to changes in D2 post-synaptic receptor sensitivity in the rat striatum. DA transporter (DAT) knockout mice exhibit increased wakefulness and less SWS. REM sleep would induce increases in dopaminergic activity after sleep deprivation and selective REM sleep deprivation for a prolonged period would result in down-regulation of DAT, enhancing dopaminergic neurotransmission. Amphetamine derivatives inhibit DAT-mediated DA reuptake [74, 75].

Short-term sleep deprivation has shown therapeutic properties for with mood disorders, long-term/ chronic sleep deprivation and disruption have instead been related to the development of mood disorders via monoamine (5-HT, NE, DA) activity dysregulation. The main symptoms of depression are due to a functional deficiency of the brain monoaminergic transmitters: norepinephrine, serotonin and/or dopamine, whereas mania is caused by a functional excess of monoamines at critical synapses in the brain. Although recently some observations have challenged the legitimacy of this theory, a dysregulation in monoamine production and transmission is still considered an important factor in the regulation of mood, emotions, cognition, motivational behaviors and stress responses. Deuschle et al. [81] conducted a study in a group of individuals suffering from chronic insomnia, and found that the short allele of the 5-HT transporter was significantly more frequent in patients suffering from insomnia than in good sleepers. Roman et al. [82] suggested that chronic sleep restriction may increase an individual's vulnerability to develop mood disorders by impairing serotoninergic transmission throughout the activation of the stress system The genetic makeup of the dopamine system involved in vulnerability to mood disorders has also been shown to be involved in the response to sleep loss and in alterations in responses to reward in humans. A polymorphism in the dopamine 2 receptor, more commonly in the dopamine transporter system, has been related to a vulnerability to psychiatric disorders in the presence of sleep deprivation in humans. It has been widely shown that individuals suffering from insomnia display hyperactivation of the hypothalamic–pituitary–adrenal-axis at both brain and peripheral levels. Increases in norepinephrine, epinephrine and other markers of sympathetic outflow have been related to cognitive and emotional arousal and somatic hyperarousal in individuals suffering from insomnia: it is the key pathophysiological mechanism of insomnia. Changes observed in brain structures in individuals suffering from insomnia include a reduction in the volume of the prefrontal cortex, caudate head and hippocampus, as well as an increase in the amygdala volume, modifications resembling those described in individuals suffering mood disorders. Given these similarities, it has been hypothesized that insomnia may influence the development and maintenance of a mood disorder throughout the activation of the stress system and of its negative consequences on the brain, including hippocampal neurogenesis, synaptic plasticity and connectivity [76–85].

Finally, we can talk about the relationship between sleep and antidepressants, which are effective on monoamine (5-HT, NE, DA) activity systems in the brain: (1) Tricyclic antidepressants (TCA) (antagonist of 5HT-1, NE, M1, H1 receptors); (a) tertiary TCAs shorten sleep latency and reduce awakenings during sleep. Therefore, it is perceived as a sedative; doxepin and amitriptyline decrease REM rate in sleep EEG, cause prolongation of REM sleep latency, (b) Secondary TCAs such as desipramine are less sedative and relatively stimulating, (c) potent serotoninergic TCAs such as clomipramine increase eye movements in NREM. It increases the periodic leg movements during sleep, (2) nonspecific reuptake inhibitors (5HT, NE DA); trazadone is sedative and nefazodone is less sedative, they increase SWS sleep, (3) monoamine oxidase inhibitors (MAOI) (eg, tranylcypromine, moclobemide), (4) selective serotonin reuptake inhibitors SSRI (eg, fluoxetine, escitalopram, paroxetine, sertraline), (5) serotonin and norepinephrine reuptake inhibitors (SNRI) (eg, venlafaxine, duloxetine, reboxetine)

(6) Bupropion (inhibition of norepinephrine and dopamine reuptake) these agents increase SWS, prolong REM latency, shorten REM time, (7) Agomelatine (agonism at melatonin M1 and M2 receptors, antagonism at serotonergic 5-HT2C receptors) have been found to increase SWS [86–89].

2.6.10 Conclusion

The more we learn about the neurophysiology of sleep and the effects of related molecules, the better we understand the pathological processes in wakefulness. Understanding the functioning of the sleep brain, along with neurotransmitters, hormones, and new molecules, will explain unknown physiological processes and inspire innovative processes in pharmacology.

Author details

Murat Kayabekir
Department of Physiology, Medical School, Atatürk University, Erzurum, Turkey

*Address all correspondence to: kayabekirmurat@gmail.com

References

[1] Guyton AC, Hall JE. Behavioral and motivational mechanisms of the brain-the limbic system and the hypothalamus. In: Textbook of Medical Physiology. 13th ed. Mississippi: Elsevier Saunders; 2011. pp. 751-761

[2] Carlson NR. Emotion. In: Physiology of Behavior. 11th ed. New Jersey: Pearson Education; 2013. pp. 361-391

[3] Carlson NR. Ingestive Behavior. In: Physiology of Behavior. 11th ed. New Jersey: Pearson Education; 2013. pp. 395-401

[4] Carlson NR. Learning and Memory. In: Physiology of Behavior. 11th ed. New Jersey: Pearson Education; 2013. pp. 437-457

[5] Kayabekir M. Sleep physiology and Polysomnogram, physiopathology and symptomatology in sleep medicine. In: Rossi FH, editor. Sleep Medicine in Clinical Neurology. 1st ed. London Bridge Street: IntechOpen; 2019. pp. 5-12

[6] Kandel ER, Schwartz JH, Jessell TM, Siegelbaum SA, Hudspeth AJ. Principles of neural science. In: Sleep and Dreaming. 5th ed. London and New York: McGraw- Hill; 2013. pp. 1140-1146. ISBN 978-0-07-139011-8

[7] Guyton AC, Hall JE. The autonomic nervous system and adrenal medulla. In: Textbook of Medical Physiology. 13th ed. Mississippi: Elsevier Saunders; 2011. pp. 773-783

[8] Kryger MH, Roth T, William CD. Normal sleep and its variations: History of sleep physiology medicine. In: Kryger MH, Roth T, William CD, editors. Principles and Practice of Sleep Medicine. 5th ed. St. Louis, Missouri: Elsevier Saunders; 2011. pp. 3-16

[9] Villablanca JR. Counterpointing the functional role of the forebrain and of the brain stem in the control of sleep-waking system. Journal of Sleep Research. 2004; 13: 179-208

[10] Kryger MH, Roth T, William CD. Sleep mechanisms and phylogeny: Neural control of sleep in mammals: Normal human sleep. In: Kryger MH, Roth T, William CD, editors. Principles and Practice of Sleep Medicine. 5th ed. Elsevier Saunders; 2011. pp. 76-80

[11] Kryger MH, Roth T, William CD. Normal sleep and its variations: Normal human sleep. In: Kryger MH, Roth T, William CD, editors. Principles and Practice of Sleep Medicine. 5th ed. St. Louis, Missouri: Elsevier Saunders; 2011. pp. 16-26

[12] Nicoll RA. Drugs that act in the central nervous system: Introduction to the Pharmacology of CNS Drugs. In: Katzung BG, Masters SB, Trevor AJ. Basic and Clinical Pharmacology. 12th ed. United States, The McGraw-Hill Companies; 2012 pp. 359-369

[13] Bush SE, Hazelwood L. 5-Hydroxytryptamine (Serotonin) and Dopamine. In: Brunton LL, Chabner BA, Knollmann BC Goodman&Gilman's The Pharmacological Basis of Therapeutics. 12th ed. United States, The McGraw-Hill Companies; 2011 pp. 335-351

[14] O' Donnell JM, Shelton RC. Drug Therapy of Depression and Anxiety Disorders. In: Brunton LL, Chabner BA, Knollmann BC Goodman&Gilman's The Pharmacological Basis of Therapeutics. 12th ed. United States, The McGraw-Hill Companies; 2011 pp. 397-413

[15] Mihic SJ, Harris RA. Hypnotics and Sedatives. In: Brunton LL, Chabner BA, Knollmann BC Goodman&Gilman's The Pharmacological Basis of Therapeutics. 12th ed. United States, The McGraw-Hill Companies; 2011 pp. 457-467

[16] Standaert DG, Roberson ED. Treatment of Central Nervous System Degenerative Disorders. In: Brunton LL, Chabner BA, Knollmann BC Goodman&Gilman's The Pharmacological Basis of Therapeutics. 12th ed. United States, The McGraw-Hill Companies; 2011 pp. 609-621

[17] Guyton AC, Hall JE. States of brain activity-sleep, brain waves, epilepsy, psychoses. In: Textbook of Medical Physiology. 13th ed. Mississippi: Elsevier Saunders; 2011. pp. 763-772

[18] Pandi-Perumal SR, Trakht I, Srinivasan V, et al. Physiological effects of melatonin: role of melatonin receptors and signal transduction pathways. Progress in Neurobiology. 2008; 85: 335-53

[19] Comai S, Gobbi G. Unveiling the role of melatonin MT2 receptors in sleep, anxiety and other neuropsychiatric diseases: a novel target in psychopharmacology. Journal of Psychiatry Neuroscience. 2014; 39: 6-21

[20] Kunz D, Schmitz S, Mahlberg R, et al. A new concept for melatonin deficit: on pineal calcification and melatonin excretion. Neuropsychopharmacology. 1999; 21: 765-772

[21] Berridge CW. Noradrenergic modulation of arousal. Brain ResearchReviews. 2008; 58: 1-7

[22] Ursin R. Seratonin and sleep. Sleep Medicine Reviews. 2002; 6:57-69

[23] Jones BE. Arousal systems. Frontiers in Bioscience. 2003; 8: 438-451

[24] Jones BE. The organization of central cholinergic systems and their functional importance in sleep-wakingstates. Progress in Brain Research. 1993; 98: 61-71

[25] Kryger MH, Roth T, William CD. Sleep mechanisms and phylogeny: Neural control of sleep in mammals: Normal human sleep. In: Kryger MH, Roth T, William CD, editors. Principles and Practice of Sleep Medicine. 5th ed. Elsevier Saunders; 2011. pp. 76-80

[26] Brainard GC, Hanifin JP. Photons, clocks, and consciousness. Journal of Biological Rhythms. 2005; 20(4): 314-325

[27] Gooley JJ, Saper CB. "Anatomy of the mammalian circadian system" In: Kryger MH, Roth T, William CD, editors. Principles and Practice of Sleep Medicine. 5th ed. Elsevier Saunders; 2011. pp. 76-80

[28] Swick TJ. The neurology of sleep. Neurologic Clinics. 2005; 23(1): 967-989

[29] Brandenberger G. The ultradian rhythm of sleep: Diverse relations with pituitary and adrenal hormones. Revista de Neurologia. 2003; 159(11): 605-610

[30] Van Cauter E, Polonsky KS, Scheen AJ. Roles of circadian rhythmicity and sleep in human glucose regulation. Endocrine Reviews. 1997; 18: 716-738

[31] Obal F Jr, Krueger JM. GHRH and sleep. Sleep Medicine Review. 2004; 8: 367-377

[32] Spiegel K, Follenius M, Simon C, et al. Prolactin secretion and sleep. Sleep. 1994; 17: 20-27

[33] Van Cauter E, Plat L, Copinschi G. Interrelations between sleep and the somatotropic axis. Sleep. 1998; 21: 553-566

[34] Holl RW, Hartmann ML, Veldhuis JD, et al. Thirty-second sampling of plasma growth hormone in man: correlation with sleep stages. Journal of Clinical Endocrinology and Metabolism. 1991: 72: 854-861

[35] Van Cauter E, Kerkhofs M, Caufriez A, et al. A quantitative

estimation of GH secretion in normal man: reproducibility and relation to sleep and time of day. Journal of Clinical Endocrinology and Metabolism. 1992; 74: 1441-1450

[36] Gronfier C, Luthringer R, Follenius M, et al. Temporal relationships between pulsatile cortisol secretion and electroencephalographic activity during sleep in man. Electroencephalogrphy Clinical Neurophysiology. 1997; 103: 405-408

[37] Pruessner JC, Wolf OT, Hellhammer DH, et al. Free cortisol levels after awakening: a reliable biological marker for the assessment of adrenocortical activity. Life Sciences. 1997; 61: 2539-2549

[38] Bierwolf C, Struve K, Marshall L, et al. Slow wave sleep drives inhibition of pituitary-adrenal secretion in humans. Journal of Neuroendocrinology. 1997; 9: 479-484

[39] Parker DC, Rossman LG, Pekary AE, et al. Effect of 64-hour sleep deprivation on the circadian waveform of thyrotropin (TSH): further evidence of sleep-related inhibition of TSH release. Journal of Clinical Endocrinology and Metabolism. 1987; 64: 157-161

[40] Brabant G, Prank K, Ranft U, et al. Physiological regulation of circadian and pulsatile thyrotropin secretion in normal man and woman. Journal of Clinical Endocrinology and Metabolism. 1990; 70: 403-409

[41] Spiegel K, Follenius M, Simon C, et al. Prolactin secretion and sleep. Sleep. 1994; 17: 20-27

[42] Van Cauter E, Copinschi G. Endocrine and other biological rhythms. DeGroot LJ Jameson JL Endocrinology. 5th ed. Philadelphia: Elsevier Saunders; 2006.pp 341-372

[43] Cauter EV, Tasali E. Endocrine Physiology in Relation to Sleep and Sleep Disturbances. In: Kryger MH, Roth T, William CD, editors. Principles and Practice of Sleep Medicine. 5th ed. Elsevier Saunders; 2011. pp. 292-300

[44] Hays J, Ockene JK, Brunner RL, et al. Effects of estrogen plus progestin on health-related quality of life. The New England Journal of Medicine: Research&Review. 2003; 348: 1839-1854

[45] Antonijevic IA, Stalla GK, Steiger A. Modulation of the sleep electroencephalogram by estrogen replacement in postmenopausal women. American Journal of Obstetrics & Gynecology. 2000; 182: 277-282

[46] Ocampo-Lim B, Guo W, DeMott Friberg R, et al. Nocturnal growth hormone (GH) secretion is eliminated by infusion of GH-releasing Hormone antagonist. Journal of Clinical Endocrinology and Metabolism. 1996; 81: 4396-4399

[47] Sakurai T: The neural circuit of orexin (hypocretin): maintaining sleep and wakefulness. Nature Review Neuroscience. 2007; 8: 171-181

[48] Ahima RS, Lazar MA: Adipokines and the peripheral and neural control of energy balance. Journal of Molecular Endochrinology. 2008; 22: 1023-1031

[49] Simon C, Gronfier C, Schlienger JL, et al.: Circadian and ultradian variations of leptin in normal man under continuous enteral nutrition: relationship to sleep and body temperature. Journal of Clinical Endocrinology and Metabolism. 1998; 83: 1893-1899

[50] Dyzma M, Boudjeltia KZ, Faraut B, Kerhofs M. Neuropeptid Y and sleep. Sleep Medicine Reviews. 2010; 14 (3): 161-165

[51] Ferreira JG, Bittencourt JC, Adamantidis A. Melanin-concentrating

hormone and sleep. Current Opinion in Neurobiology. 2017; 44: 152-158

[52] Bittencourt JC. Anatomical organization of the melanin-concentrating hormone peptide family in the mammalian brain. General and Comparative Endocrinology. 2011; 172 (2): 185-197

[53] Nishino S, Kanbayashi T: Symptomatic narcolepsy, cataplexy and hypersomnia, and their implications in the hypothalamic hypocretin/orexin system. Sleep Medicine Review. 2005; 9: 269-310

[54] Kemp EH, Weetman AP. Melanin-concentrating hormone and melanin-concentrating hormone receptors in mammalian skin physiopathology. Peptides. 2009; 30 (11): 2071-2075

[55] Lydic R, Baghdoyan HA, McGinley J. Opioids, sedation and sleep. Different states, similar traits, and the search for common mechanisms. In: Malviya S, Naughton N, Tremper KK editors. Contemporary Clinical Neuroscience: Sedation and Analgesia for Diagnostic and Therapeutic Procedures. Humana Press, Totowa, NJ; 2003. pp 1-31

[56] Nelson LE, Guo TZ, Saper CB, Franks NP, Maze M. The sedative component of anesthesia is mediated by GABAa receptors in an endogenous sleep pathway. Nature Neurosciense. 2002; 5: 979-984

[57] Lin JS, Hou Y, Sakai K, Jouvet M. Histaminergic descending inputs to the mesopontine tegmentum and their role in the control of cortical activation and wakefulness in the cat. Journal of Neuroscience. 1996; 16:1523-1537

[58] Benowitz NL. Pharmacology of nicotine: addiction and therapeutics. Annual Review Pharmacologyl Toxicology. 1996; 36: 597-613

[59] Hughes JR, Hatsukami DK, Mitchell JE, Dahlgren LA. Prevalence of smoking among psychiatric outpatients. American Journal of Psychology. 1996: 143; 993-997

[60] Seiden LS, Lew R, Malberg JE. Neurotoxicity of methamphetamine and methylenedioxymethamphetamine. Neurotoxicity Research. 2001; 3: 101-116

[61] Seiden LS, Sabol KE. Amphetamine: effects on catecholamine systems and behavior. Annual Review Pharmacology Toxicology. 1993; 32: 639-677

[62] Ferraro L, Antonelli T, Taganelli S, et al. The vigilance promoting drug modafinil increases extracellular glutamate levels in the medial preoptic area and the posterior hypothalamus of the conscious rat: prevention by local GABAa receptor blockade. Neuropsychopharmacology. 1999; 20: 346-356

[63] Garcia-Rill E, Biedermann JA, Chambers T, Skinner RD, Mrak RE, Husain M, Karson CN. Mesopontine neurons in schizophrenia. Neuroscience. 1995; 66: 321-335

[64] Qureshi A, Lee-Chiong T. Medications and their effects on sleep. Medical Clinics North America. 2004; 88: 751-766

[65] Boutros NN, Mucci A, Vignapiano A, Galderisi S. Electrophysiological Aberrations Associated with Negative Symptoms in Schizophrenia. Curr Top Behav Neurosci. 2014; 21: 129-156

[66] Fermin, A. M., Afzal, U., & Culebras, A. Sleep in Neuromuscular Diseases. Sleep Medicine Clinics. 2016; 11: 53-64

[67] Brown RH, Al-Chalabi M. Amyotrophic lateral sclerosis. The New

England Journal of Medicine. 2017; 377: 162-172

[68] Stochi F, Barbato L, Nordera G, Barardelli A, Ruggieri S. Sleep disorders in Parkinson' s disease. Journal of Neurology. 1998; 245: 5-8

[69] Dauvilliers Y, Mayer G, Lecendreux M, Neidhart E, Peraita-Adrados R, Sonka K, Biliard M, Tafti M. Kleine–Levin syndrome. An autoimmune hypothesis based on clinical and genetic analyses. Neurology. 2002; 59: 1739-1745

[70] Garcia-Rill E. Disorders of the reticular activating system. Medical Hypothesis. 1997; 49: 379-387

[71] Maquet P. Positron emission tomography studies of sleep and sleep disorders. Journal of Neurology. 1997; 244: 23-28

[72] Scheen AJ, Byrne MM, Plat L, Van Cauter E. Relationships between sleep quality and glucose regulation in normal humans. American Journal of Physiology. 1996; 271: 261-270

[73] Spiegel K, Leproult R, L'Hermite-Baleriaux M, Copinschi G, Penev PD, Van Cauter E. Leptin levels are dependent on sleep duration: relationships with sympathovagal balance, carbohydrate regulation, cortisol, and thyrotropin. Journal of Clinical Endocrinology and Metabolism. 2004; 89: 5762-5771

[74] Lammers CH, D'Souza U, Qin ZH, Lee SH, Yajima S, Mouradian MM. Regulation of striatal dopamine receptors by estrogen. Synapse. 1999; 34: 222-227

[75] Lima MM, Andersen ML, Reksidler AB, et al. Blockage of dopaminergic D (2) receptors produces decrease of REM but not of slow wave sleep in rats after REM sleep deprivation. Behavioral Brain Research. 2008; 188: 406-411

[76] Adrien, J. Neurobiological bases for the relation between sleep and depression. Sleep Medicine Reviews. 2002; 6: 341-351

[77] Muneer, A. The neurobiology of bipolar disorder: An integrated approach. Chonnam Medical Journal. 2016; 52: 18-37

[78] aan het Rot M, Mathew SJ, & Charney DS. Neurobiological mechanisms in major depressive disorder. Canadian Medical Association Journal. 2009; 180: 305-313

[79] Ruhe HG, Mason NS, & Schene AH. Mood is indirectly related to serotonin, norepinephrine and dopamine levels in humans: A meta-analysis of monoamine depletion studies. Molecular Psychiatry. 2007; 12: 331-359

[80] Chaudhury D, Liu H, & Han MH. Neuronal correlates of depression. Cellular and Molecular Life Sciences. 2015; 72: 4825-4848

[81] Deuschle M, Schredl M, Schilling C, Wüst S, Frank J, Witt SH, Schulze TG. Association between a serotonin transporter length polymorphism and primary insomnia. Sleep. 2010; 33: 343-347

[82] Roman V, Walstra I, Luiten PG, & Meerlo P. Too little sleep gradually desensitizes the serotonin 1A receptor system. Sleep. 2005; 28:1505-1510

[83] Holst SC, Muller T, Valomon A, Seebauer B, Berger W & Landolt HP. Functional polymorphisms in dopaminergic genes modulate neurobehavioral and neurophysiological consequences of sleep deprivation. Scientific Reports. 2017; 745-982

[84] Morin CM, Drake CL, Harvey AG, Krystal AD, Manber R, Riemann D &

Spiegelhalder K. Insomnia disorder. Nature Reviews. Disease Primers. 2017; 1: 15-26

[85] Riemann D, Nissen C, Palagini L, Otte A, Perlis ML & Spiegelhalder K. The neurobiology, investigation, and treatment of chronic insomnia. The Lancet Neurology. 2015; 14: 547-558

[86] Wichniak A, Wierzbicka A, Jernajczyk W. Sleep and antidepressant treatment. Current Pharmaceutical Design. 2012; 18: 5802-5817

[87] Thompson C. Onset of action of antidepressants: results of different analyses. Human Psychopharmacology. 2002; 17(1): 27-32

[88] Jindal RD, Friedman ES, Berman SR, Fasiczka AL, Howland RH, Thase ME. Effects of sertraline on sleep architecture in patients with depression. Journal Clinical Psychopharmacology. 2003; 23: 540-548

[89] Hickie IB, Rogers NL. Novel melatonin-based therapies: potential advances in the treatment of major depression. Lancet. 2011; 378: 621-631

Section 2

Pharmacotherapy in Sleep Disorders

Chapter 3

Narcolepsy Treatment: Present and Future

Juan José Ortega-Albás, Raquel López García, Alfonso Martínez Martínez, Sonia Carratalá Monfort, Juan Antonio Royo Prats, Laura Albiol Varela and Patricia Ortega Gabás

Abstract

Narcolepsy is a chronic, disabling sleep disorder with a significant diagnostic delay. Nowadays, treatment is focused on managing symptoms that impacts patient's life, such as at workplace, social events or even at school, but not aimed cure the disease. However, we have pharmacological treatments that effectively help control the main symptoms (excessive daytime sleepiness, cataplexy, fragmentation of nocturnal sleep, sleep paralysis and hypnagogic and hypnopompic hallucinations). On the other hand, pharmacological treatment must be individualised as there are great variations in severity, order of appearance symptoms and development of the disease. We intend to expose the different symptomatic treatments recommended by clinical guidelines and the clinical management from a practical point of view. Future treatments include therapies based on the replacement of hypocretin or the administration of agonist receptors. Other techniques such as hypothalamic stem cell transplantation, gene replacement therapy or immunotherapy are also being investigated.

Keywords: narcolepsy, sleep, cataplexy, pharmacotherapy, pharmacology, sleepiness

1. Introduction

Narcolepsy is a chronic and disabling disease, which, according to the International Classification of Sleep Disorders (ICSD-3), considered to be hypersomnias of central origin [1]. Narcolepsy presents with a variable combination of sleep–wake symtoms and motor, psychiatric, emotional, cognitive, metabolic and autonomic disturbances that reflect the hypothalamic origin of the disorder.

The leading symptoms are:

1. Excessive daytime sleepiness (EDS), which can also manifest with sleep attacks, involuntary napping, automatic behaviours, difficulty sustaining attention and memory disturbances.

2. Cataplexy, briefs episodes of bilateral loss of muscle tone triggered by sudden emotions in the presence of a normal state of consciousness. Often is partial, rarely complete with falls.

Other sleep–wake symptoms are fatigue, sleep paralysis, hypnagogic and hypnopompic hallucinations, nightmares, lucid dreams, enacted dreams, disrupted night-time sleep, restless legs syndrome or parasomnias.

The current International Classification of Sleep Disorders (ICSD-3) defines two types of narcolepsy:

a. Narcolepsy type 1 (NT1): EDS for > 3 months in association with either CSF orexin levels < 110 pg./ml or cataplexy and a mean sleep latency < 8 minutes on the multiple sleep latency test (MSLT) and at least two sleep onset REM periods (SOREMPs) during MSLT y/o night-time polysomnography.

b. Narcolepsy type 2 (NT2): EDS for > 3 months in the absence of cataplexy but with a mean sleep latency on the MSLT < 8 minutes and at least two SOREMPs on the MSLT y/o night-time polysomnography, as well as CSF orexin levels > 110 pg./ml (or not measured).

If cataplexy develops over time or CSF orexin levels decrease to < 110 pg./ml, the diagnosis of NT2 must be change to NT1.

The main symptoms of NT1 are related to hypocretin/orexin (ORX) deficiency, due to the selective destruction, likely autoimmune in origin, of ORX-producing hypothalamic neurons. Likewise, hypocretin deficiency reduces the excitatory signal of the neurons responsible for the synthesis of neurotransmitters that promote wakefulness, such as noradrenaline (NA), dopamine (DA), serotonin (5-HT) and histamine.

Genetically, approximately 98% of patients with NT1 carry the HLA class II allele DQB1*06:02; this allele is present in 50% of patients with NT2 and only 12–30% of the general population [2]. So far, no specific antibodies against ORX neurons have been detected. This could be due either to their location in a restricted area where there is a small number of damaged antibodies, or because the activation of specific T cells is negligible.

There is a clear variability in the evolution of the disease over time. On one hand, it is important to note that when a patient develops symptoms, the hypocretinergic neurons may already present irreversible damage; on the other hand, on average, there is a diagnostic delay of 10 years from the onset of symptoms. For this reason, it is still not possible to establish a concrete and extrapolable pattern. Some patients observed with severe narcolepsy and cataplexy show full symptomatology in the first days of the disease, while others develop a progressive course with excessive daytime sleepiness (EDS) as the initial symptom and followed by cataplexy after months or years of evolution.

Different hypotheses have been postulated regarding the pathophysiology of cataplexy. On one hand, there is a direct relationship between the brain areas responsible for inhibition of muscle tone in REM sleep and hypocretinergic neurons. The loss of these neurons would cause dissociated REM sleep (the atonia of the REM phase would appear during wakefulness) manifesting itself clinically as cataplexy or sleep paralysis [3]. Likewise, it has been proposed that hypocretin deficiency would facilitate sleep–wake transitions more frequently due to the instability of wake–sleep regulation mechanisms.

Pharmacotherapy in the treatment of narcolepsy is currently aimed at controlling the principal symptoms: EDS, cataplexy, sleep fragmentation, sleep paralysis and hypnagogic and hypnopompic hallucinations, but are not intended to cure the disease. However, the treatment does manage to significantly improve quality of life.

The following is a detailed breakdown of the different existing treatments and the promising future lines that are being developed for the treatment of Narcolepsy.

2. Existing lines of therapy

As we have already mentioned, current therapies are aimed at the symptomatic treatment of narcolepsy. One key point to take into account is the high degree of inter-individual variability in the clinical presentation of the disease, in terms of the different clinical evolution over the years, and the therapeutic response and possible side effects related to the different treatments.

The first approach should therefore focus on the adoption of non-pharmacological measures, with programmed short-duration daytime naps being one of the most prominent.

Establishment of rigid schedules for waking up and going to bed, attempting to avoid transgressions or sleep deprivation, should be recommended. Like other patients with sleep disorders, avoiding excessive caffeine or alcohol consumption should be recommended. Last, but not least, it is helpful to orient the patient from the point of view of work, providing suggestions as to the jobs that are most advisable and less advisable for patients with narcolepsy. In addition, they should be informed of associations or support groups at the national and international level.

Regarding pharmacological therapy, the different existing lines of therapy can be classified according to their mode of action or according to the type of symptomatology that they are intended to treat (daytime sleepiness, cataplexy, sleep fragmentation, etc.).

2.1 Recommended treatments for excessive daytime sleepiness (EDS)

1. Modafinil: inhibits the dopamine transporter, facilitating an increase in its concentration, although its mechanism of action is still unclear. Approved by the FDA and EMA. Armodafinil is also FDA approved and the usual doses for adults range from 100 to 250 mg.

   Dosage: in tablets of 100–400 mg orally. Initially, treatment is started with 100 mg, which can be divided into two intakes of 50 mg at least 2 hours apart. The dose should later be increased depending on the degree of drowsiness, considering the dose-dependent occurrence of side effects.

   Pharmacokinetics: the absorption of modafinil is fast, with a maximum plasma concentration of about 2 to 4 h. The effective elimination half-life of modafinil after multiple doses is approximately 15 h. The main route of excretion is via the liver and part of its metabolites via the kidneys. Patients with severe hepatic impairment should be treated with lower doses. Reversible inhibition of the cytochrome P450 enzyme CYP2C19, as well as CYP3A4, CYP1A2 and CYP2B633 has been observed. Coadministration of modafinil with diazepam, phenytoin and propranolol, which are eliminated via the CYP2C19 enzyme, may increase their levels. It is recommended that alternative methods of contraception be considered during treatment with modafinil and one month after the end of the treatment.

   Safety and adverse events: generally well tolerated and the most common adverse events were headache (13%), nervousness (8%) and nausea (5%). Treatment-related cardiovascular events were infrequent, including palpitations (1.5%), hypertension (1%) and tachycardia (1%). Studies with modafinil have shown a potential for dependence, so the possibility of dependence with long-term use cannot be completely ruled out. It is also recommended that an ECG be performed on all patients prior to the start of treatment.

The combination of modafinil with connexin-30 inhibitors is under development (discussed later in the chapter).

2. Methylphenidate: blocks the reuptake of noradrenaline and dopamine (inhibiting the transporters of these neurotransmitters at the presynaptic level) increasing the concentration of dopamine and noradrenaline in the synaptic cleft. Broadly speaking, this generates its stimulant effect within the central nervous system (CNS), primarily in the prefrontal cortex. It is also a weak agonist at the 5-HT1A receptor, which is an additional mechanism that contributes to increased dopamine levels. Before starting any treatment with stimulants, it is advisable to perform at least an electrocardiogram to rule out possible cardiac arrhythmias [4]. Due to the risk of serious side effects, avoiding use with patients with structural heart abnormalities is recommended.

   Dosage: doses are administered orally and range between 10 and 60 mg and should not exceed 72 mg. Immediate and extended release are available.

   Adverse effects: insomnia and nervousness are the most frequent events, although other effects related to the CNS (dizziness, headache, tics, akathisia), gastrointestinal (nausea/vomiting, dry mouth, decreased appetite, weight loss, abdominal pain) and cardiovascular system (tachycardia and palpitations) have also been reported. Methylphenidate is FDA approved for the treatment of attention deficit hyperactivity disorder (ADHD) in children and adults and as a second-line treatment for narcolepsy in adults.

3. Pitolisant: histamine H3-receptor antagonist-inverse agonist (to be developed later).

4. Amphetamines or dextroamphetamine: the main action is through increases in synaptic concentrations of monoamine neurotransmitters, thus indirectly enhancing noradrenergic and dopaminergic neurotransmission in the CNS. Catecholaminergic signalling is the primary mediator of efficacy in narcolepsy. This same pathway is also responsible for the major side effects, as well as its potential for abuse. It should be considered that it is a drug with very limited use, because there is a difficult balance between achieving correct therapeutic efficacy and an acceptable control of side effects.

   Dosage: doses between 5 and 30 mg orally, twice a day, or 20 mg in a sustained release formulation twice a day are usually used.

   Adverse effects: decreased appetite, nausea, vomiting, insomnia, headache, increased blood pressure and heart rate, etc.

   Safety: has a high potential for abuse, can cause psychosis and manic episodes.

2.2 Recommended treatments for cataplexy and symptoms resulting from dysregulation of REM sleep

1. Sodium oxybate (Xyrem®): this is the sodium salt of gamma-hydroxybutyrate (GHB). GHB is synthesised in neurons throughout the CNS and is an active metabolite of gamma-aminobutyric acid (GABA). It inhibits noradrenergic neurons in the locus coeruleus during sleep, with a rebound effect of these neurons during the day thus promoting wakefulness, although its mechanism of action remains unclear. One of the hypotheses about the mechanism of action on the control of EDS and cataplexy postulates that it could be mediated

through GABA-B agonist actions on dopaminergic, noradrenergic, as well as thalamocortical neurons. In 1998, the FDA granted permission to test oxybate as an orphan drug for narcolepsy. In 2002 it developed a distribution program through hospital pharmacies only. And in Europe, it is available under restricted prescription and special situation. It also has a risk management and pharmacovigilance program.

Dosage: it is an oral solution (500 mg/ml). The recommended initial dose is 4.5 g/night (divided into 2 doses, each of 2.25 grams) spaced at least 2.5–4 hours apart before the new dose, so that most of the drug has been eliminated when the patient wakes up. Up to a maximum of 9 g/day (7 g/day in children <12 years).

Pharmacokinetics: it is rapidly absorbed with a maximum plasma concentration (tmax) of 1.5–2 h. Less than 5% of the unaltered drug appears in the urine 6–8 h after dosing. No active metabolites. Also does not induce cytochrome P450 enzymes. In patients with cirrhosis of the liver, a lower dose should be started because a doubling of the area under the curve, reduced oral clearance and prolonged elimination half-life have been observed.

Safety: the most frequent adverse effects were: headache (11.6%), nasopharyngitis (6.4%), dizziness (5.2%), weight loss (5.2%), nausea (5.1%), urinary incontinence in (2.4%) and sleepwalking in (3.1%). Serious adverse events included depression, angina, inguinal hernia, psychosis or attempted suicide. In addition, the European Medicines Agency (EMA) recommends assessing the risk/benefit in patients with obstructive sleep apnoea syndrome (OSA), especially in doses higher than 6 g/night. On the other hand, it is important to control daily salt intake in patients with heart failure, hypertension or renal failure because the molecule has a high salt content. It also must be taken under consideration the potential for abuse, before being administered, the patient's medical history should be reviewed.

Recently, a multi-centre, randomised, placebo-controlled trial involving children and adolescents with narcolepsy with cataplexy was developed examining efficacy and safety. Based on this study, the FDA approved the use of sodium oxybate in paediatric patients with narcolepsy beginning at seven years of age.

There are now new therapeutic lines with controlled-release GHB (see below).

2. Pitolisant: histamine H3-receptor inverse antagonist–agonist (to be developed later).

3. Venlafaxine and Duloxetine: are dual serotonin and noradrenaline reuptake inhibitors. These are the most used antidepressants to control cataplexy. This recommendation lacks clinical evidence of efficacy and is based solely on expert opinions.

   Dosage: initially 37.5 mg, sometimes requiring higher doses (75–300 mg). The extended-release form is preferable.

   Safety: It can be administered to children and is not recommended for pregnant women.

4. Fluoxetine and Citalopram: are selective serotonin reuptake inhibitors (SSRIs). A crossover study comparing clomipramine and fluvoxamine showed that

SSRIs improved cataplexy, but were less active than the antidepressant. Studies have been carried out with femoxetine, zimelidine and escitalopram showing a clear anticataplectic effect and good tolerance.

5. Reboxetine: dopamine and noradrenaline reuptake inhibitor (discussed below).

6. Monoamine oxidase inhibitors (MAOIs): act by inhibiting the enzyme monoamine oxidase by increasing the availability of monoamine neurotransmitters. A suppression of REM sleep has been observed as the main effect. Phenelzine has been used successfully in seven patients with resistant narcolepsy, with persistent efficacy after 1 year of treatment. In addition, there have been two placebo-controlled studies with selegiline (MAO-B inhibitors) at doses of 20–40 mg which demonstrated a significant reduction in the frequency of cataplexy. With MAO-A inhibitors such as brofaromine, significant results were also obtained, reducing cataplexy with no significant side effects. However, they are rarely used in clinical practice due to their adverse effects (weight gain, orthostatic hypotension, irritability, sweating, dry mouth, etc.)

7. Tricyclic antidepressants (TCAs): are non-specific monoamine reuptake inhibitors that increase the availability of serotonin, noradrenaline and dopamine. Some also have anticholinergic effects that may affect the anti-cataplegic properties.

   Dosage: between 10 and 150 mg, generally lower doses than those used as an antidepressant are needed to be effective in controlling cataplexy and its effects are very fast (only a few days) compared to the effects as an antidepressant. Several antidepressants have been tried, but clomipramine has been the most commonly used TCA.

   Safety: if the antidepressant is abruptly discontinued, an elevated risk of rebound cataplexy or "status cataplecticus" has been observed.

It should be noted that the Class I evidence for Narcolepsy with cataplexy (NT1) and without cataplexy (NT2) was obtained for the previously described psychostimulant drugs and for sodium oxybate. Oxybate therefore remains the first-line treatment of choice in NT1, especially for the control of cataplexy, although as we will see below, pitolisant demonstrated efficacy similar to oxybate in patients with NT1 in a recent randomised placebo-controlled clinical trial.

2.3 Treatments currently being developed

1. Pitolisant (Wakix®): as we have explained previously, this is an inverse agonist of the histamine H3 receptor (competitive H3R antagonist) that acts at presynaptic level activating histaminergic neurons (it blocks the inhibitory effect of histamine on the release of endogenous histamine and improves the release in the entire central nervous system) favouring wakefulness and also with an additive anticataplectic effect. It was designated an Orphan Medicinal Product by the European Medicines Agency in 2007 and confirmed again in 2016 [5]. It was also granted orphan drug status by the FDA in 2010. It has been approved by the European Medicines Agency (EMA) in 2016 and by the FDA in 2019 for NT1 and NT2.

Dosage: single morning dose (9–36 mg/day) orally. 4.5 mg and 18 mg tablets. In Spain it is dispensed in hospital pharmacies. The guideline approved in Europe is as follows:

1st week: the starting dose is 9 mg divided into two 4.5 mg tablets to be administered at the same time in the morning.

2nd week: increase to one 18 mg tablet or consider decreasing the dose to 4.5 mg.

3rd week: the recommended dose is 36 mg, consisting of two 18 mg tablets.

Pharmacokinetics: it is rapidly absorbed, with a maximum plasma concentration (tmax) of 3.5 h and an elimination half-life (t1/2) of approximately 10–12 hours. It is metabolised through cytochrome p450 (CYP3A4) and (CYP2D6) and eliminated in urine as inactive metabolites and 25% of the dose is excreted through exhaled air.

Safety: it has a good tolerance profile even after one year of follow-up, as well as good control of cataplexy. It should be noted that Pitolisant would be of special interest to patients with cardiovascular comorbidities. It has very low abuse potential: a study in comparison to Phentermine and a placebo in patients with a history of recreational polydrug use indicated that Pitolisant, at therapeutic and supratherapeutic doses, has a similar abuse risk to the placebo. The maximum recommended dose in moderate–severe hepatic or renal impairment is 17.8 mg and it is contraindicated in end-stage kidney disease or severe liver disease. In women of childbearing age, it is recommended that a non-hormonal method of contraception be used during treatment and 21 days after stopping treatment. Antidepressants and antihistamines (which cross the blood–brain barrier) may reduce the efficacy of Pitolisant and special caution should be exercised because of the narrow therapeutic margin when using certain treatments such as immunosuppressants.

In a clinical trial, it was observed that pitolisant did not modify the pharmacokinetic profiles of oxybate or modafinil, and oxybate showed no relevant effect on pitolisant. However, a reduction in exposure was observed with modafinil, although no dose adjustment was necessary.

Side effects: in order of frequency were insomnia (8.4%), headache (7.7%), nausea (4.8%), anxiety (2.1%), irritability (1.8%), dizziness, etc. The most serious adverse effects: abnormal weight loss and miscarriage (only 0.09%).

In the HAROSA I and II trials in patients with Obstructive Sleep Apnoea Syndrome and cardiovascular comorbidities, no changes in systolic and diastolic blood pressure and heart rate were observed [6] compared to a placebo. Supratherapeutic doses between 108 and 216 mg produce an increase in the QTc interval (10–13 ms), so caution should be exercised with those drugs that prolong QT. No ECG is required before starting treatment.

Based on our clinical experience in the Sleep Unit of the Hospital General Universitario de Castellón, below we provide the results of patients who followed the compassionate-use program prior to commercialization, to initiate treatment with pitolisant in 14 adult patients and one patient with paediatric narcolepsy who did not respond to the treatments available at that time:

8 patients diagnosed with NT1: request made on the basis of EDS, and/or persistent cataplexy.

Resistance or intolerance to available treatments (modafinil, sodium oxybate, dimethylphenidate ...)

3 patients with NT2: two patients with secondary narcolepsy (Steinert's myotonic dystrophy, Devic's neuromyelitis optica) and one patient with intolerance to modafinil and/or dimethylphenidate.

2 patients with idiopathic hypersomnia: one patient who reported severe hypersomnia and another patient in whom Modafinil was contraindicated due to adverse effects.

1 patient with obstructive sleep apnoea syndrome (OSAHS) who presented residual hypersomnolence without improvement with modafinil.

A 14-year-old boy with narcolepsy without cataplexy, as first line treatment for excessive daytime sleepiness after having been treated with methylphenidate.

Currently, all patients with NT2, idiopathic hypersomnia and sleepiness secondary to (OSA) continue to be treated and the symptoms of EDS have been corrected.

Of the patients with NT1, 3 continue to be treated and the cataplexy, which was mild–moderate, has been controlled. The other 5 patients dropped out due to lack of response because they presented severe cataplexy since being diagnosed with the disease.

In Ref. to safety and adverse events (AE): 2 patients out of the 15 who started treatment with pitolisant had conciliation insomnia. One was a patient with NT2 secondary to neuromyelitis optica, who presented this symptomatology with a dose of 18 mg, which was resolved by lowering the dose to 13.5 mg. The second patient presented NT1, in treatment with sodium oxybate 5.5 grams/night associated with pitolisant 36 mg/day that reverted when the dose of pitolisant was reduced to 22.5 mg. There was no other type of AE.

2. Solriamfetol (JZP-110): a selective dopamine and noradrenaline reuptake inhibitor (with no effect on the release of other monoamines) intended to improve drowsiness (EDS) in patients with obstructive sleep apnoea or narcolepsy [7]. In 2019, the FDA approved it for narcolepsy-associated drowsiness and the EMA is currently reviewing the marketing authorisation application for this indication. At the moment, experience with Solriamfetol is limited.

   Dose: range 75–150 mg/day of oral administration.

   Pharmacokinetics: it is rapidly absorbed, with a maximum plasma concentration (tmax) of 2 hours and an elimination half-life (t1/2) of approximately 7 hours. It is minimally metabolised and excreted mainly in the urine as an unchanged drug. Dose adjustment is recommended in moderate and severe renal insufficiency (maximum doses 75 and 37.5 mg/day, respectively). It should not be used concomitantly with monoamine oxidase inhibitors (MAOIs), which should be discontinued 2 weeks in advance.

   Adverse events: headache (11.1%), nausea (6.6%) and decreased appetite (6.8%) and less frequently dry mouth, constipation, anxiety and palpitations.

It is important to note that it is not necessary to discontinue oral and hormonal contraception as is recommended for modafinil and pitolisant.

Safety: Abuse potential was assessed in patients with a history of recreational polydrug use compared to phentermine. In conclusion, they present a similar or lower risk of abuse than phentermine and have therefore received a Schedule IV designation in the United States.

Two studies have been conducted: a first 12-week, randomised, double-blind, placebo-controlled phase IIb trial to evaluate efficacy in adults with narcolepsy with or without cataplexy. And a similarly designed phase III trial of 12 weeks duration for the treatment of obstructive sleep apnoea and EDS in narcolepsy.

3. Summary

In recent years there has been a significant increase in new therapeutic options such as Pitolisant and Solriamfetol, aimed at developing better control of narcolepsy symptoms.

Pitolisant is positioned as a first-line drug of choice for the management of symptoms such as excessive daytime sleepiness and cataplexy, in addition to being able to be used in both adults and children, and is the only one of the new therapeutic lines whose use is considered in paediatric narcolepsy. With regard to the usual treatments, as we have already mentioned, a clinical trial with sodium oxybate in the paediatric population has also been published recently.

Solriamfetol would be included in the first line treatment of excessive daytime sleepiness (EDS) in adults. In addition, the use of both Pitolisant and Solriamfetol would be advisable as a first-line strategy, in combination with the other anticataplectic drugs for a better control of cataplexy. Both can be used in combination for second-line treatment of EDS.

Pharmacological strategy of the European guidelines for the treatment of narcolepsy [8]:

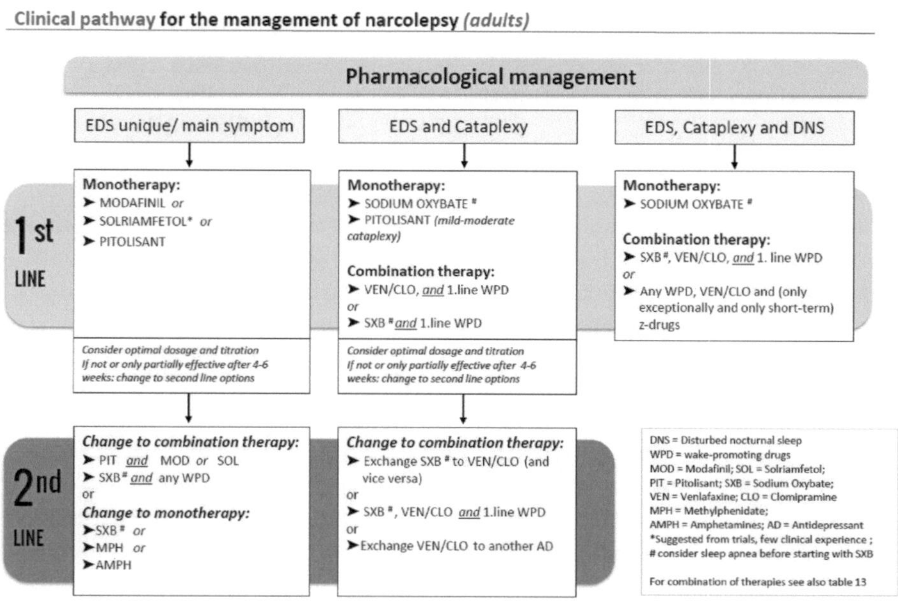

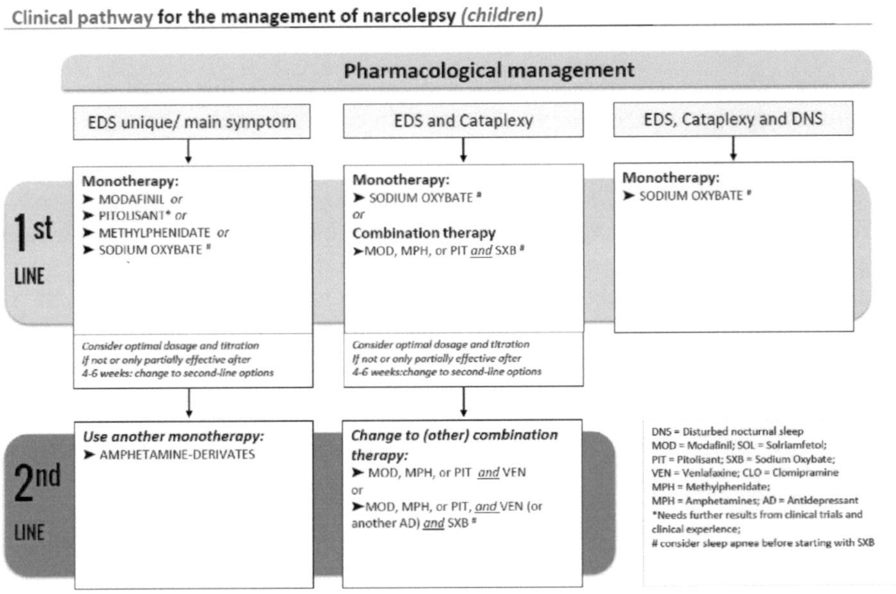

3.1 Therapies under development

1. AXS-12 (Reboxetine): a selective NA reuptake inhibitor with a weak effect on 5-HT reuptake and no effect on DA reuptake. It is a drug initially intended for the treatment of depression. It is currently in development for the treatment of cataplexy and EDS associated with narcolepsy. The FDA has designated it as an orphan drug. Preclinical data have shown a reduction in cataplexy and sleep attacks in narcoleptic mice (attributed to an effect on NA reuptake inhibition). Since noradrenaline reuptake inhibitors are very effective for the treatment of cataplexy, it will probably be used to control cataplexy and become an alternative for patients who cannot take oxybate and pitolisant. One of the possible indications could be the treatment of patients with major depressive disorder and narcolepsy [8].

   Pharmacokinetics: Rapidly absorbed after oral administration (tmax) approximately 2–4 h and eliminated mainly through metabolism by CYP3A4.

   Safety: A Phase II, randomised, double-blind, placebo-controlled, crossover study is underway in participants with narcolepsy with cataplexy and EDS.

   Adverse events: dry mouth, hyperhidrosis, constipation and restlessness were reported in a 2-week pilot study. Post-marketing experience (with indication for depression) has reported other AEs such as: insomnia, dizziness, dry mouth, constipation, nausea and hyperhidrosis.

2. THN102 (modafinil/flecainide): this is the association of the inhibitory effect of astroglial connexins associated with a dopamine reuptake inhibitor, improving the coupling of astroglial cells, since it is believed that astrocytes and astroglial connexins are involved in the regulation of sleep and wakefulness. In the cortex, modafinil would act by increasing the expression of messenger RNA (mRNA) and the connexin 30 protein, one of the main astroglial connections. On the other hand, flecainide has an inhibitory effect on astroglial connexins. In preclinical studies, flecainide enhanced the

procognitive and wakefulness-promoting effects of modafinil in mice and modafinil/flecainide coadministration decreased the number and duration of direct transitions to REM sleep in orexin-inactivated mice.

Pharmacokinetics: not specifically reported. Data from mouse models indicate that flecainide did not affect the pharmacokinetic parameters and bioavailability of modafinil.

Efficacy: evaluated in a three-way, phase II, double-blind, randomised, placebo-controlled, crossover trial in 48 adults with narcolepsy with or without cataplexy for 2 weeks. Participants received modafinil/flecainide 300/3 mg, modafinil/flecainide 300/27 mg and modafinil 300 mg/placebo in each of the three periods. Preliminary results indicated no difference in efficacy between THN102 and modafinil alone. This could be due to an over-representation of participants with severe narcolepsy who presented a low response to modafinil.

Safety: no safety data currently available.

The potential role of THN102 in narcolepsy is unclear. The narcolepsy study was stopped due to lack of efficacy in the phase II study.

3. Divalproex sodium: increases exposure to sodium oxybate, allowing the dose of sodium oxybate to be decreased. Concomitant use of other central nervous system (CNS) depressants may intensify the central depressant effects of sodium oxybate.

4. FT-218: (Controlled-release sodium oxybate): acts on the GABA-B agonist receptors and uses Micropump technology®, a microparticle platform that can be used to achieve prolonged or delayed delivery of orally administered small-molecule drugs. The dosage would therefore be only once a night. The FDA has currently designated it as an orphan drug.

   Dosage: 4.5–6-7.5 or 9 g once a night.

   Pharmacokinetics: A Phase III trial evaluating the bioavailability of FT218 compared to immediate-release sodium oxybate (Xyrem®) in healthy volunteers is currently under development.

   Efficacy: of FT218 is being evaluated in another phase III, multi-centre, double-blind, placebo-controlled REST-ON trial (Randomised study Evaluating the efficacy and SafeTy of a Once Nightly formulation of sodium oxybate). Adverse effects are expected to be similar to immediate-release sodium oxybate.

5. JZP-258: is a new low sodium oxybate product (combination of sodium oxybate, potassium oxybate, calcium oxybate and magnesium oxybate) and has 92% less sodium. It would therefore be more advisable for use in patients with hypertension, heart failure or renal failure). In addition, it is tolerated better because it does not leave an unpleasant taste and does not have as many gastrointestinal effects as sodium oxybate.

   Pharmacokinetics: lower Cmax, longer tmax and similar AUC were obtained compared to sodium oxybate.

   Efficacy: evaluated in a phase III multi-centre, randomised, phase III withdrawal study.

Adverse events: reported most frequently were headache (22.4%), nausea (13.4%) and dizziness (11.4%); treatment-related SAEs were reported in only two participants. In addition, a 24-week open-label safety study is underway.

6. SUVN-G3031: is an inverse agonist of the histamine 3 receptor (H3R) that is in phase II development.

   Anticataplectic and wakefulness-promoting effects have been observed in rodents, increasing acetylcholine, histamine, DA and NA levels in the cortex, but without altering DA levels in the striatum or nucleus accumbens, which might suggest a lower abuse potential. No adverse effects on ECG parameters, fertility, embryofoetal development or CNS safety concerns have been reported in preclinical studies.

7. TAK-925: is a selective agonist of the hypocretin/orexin 2 receptor (ORX2R). It has demonstrated wakefulness-promoting effects in wild mice and primates. It also increased wakefulness time and improved wakefulness fragmentation and cataplexy and attenuated weight gain in ORX/ataxin-3 transgenic mice without changing food intake. If the results are confirmed, it could be targeted to treat a wide range of symptoms without causing ORX2R desensitisation.

   Pharmacokinetics: A Phase I study with single ascending doses (7–240 mg, administered as an intravenous infusion over 9 hours) has been conducted in 36 healthy volunteers, evaluating safety, pharmacokinetics and tolerability. In addition, another placebo-controlled crossover study was carried out in 14 NT1 patients where doses of (5, 11.2 and 44.8 mg, as a 9 h intravenous infusion) were administered [9]. The exposure was proportional to the dose over the dose range studied and t1/2 was less than 2 h; PKs were similar in healthy volunteers and NT1 patients.

   Adverse events: increase in blood pressure and HR. Improved mean sleep latency as determined by the TMW maintenance of wakefulness test in NT1 patients (from 22.4, 37.6, and 40.0 min with TAK-925 5, 11.2, and 44.8 mg, respectively, compared to 2.9 min with placebo.

8. TAK-994a selective hypocretin/orexin 2 receptor agonist (administered orally), has been shown to increase wakefulness and reduce cataplexy-like episodes in mouse models and to improve wakefulness fragmentation in these models.

4. Future therapies

A. Administration of orexin peptides (ORXR2) as effective stimulants may also be of interest to decrease EDS in patients with NT2 and idiopathic hypersomnia and associated conditions with normal CSF ORX levels.

B. Neural transplantation of orexin: Hypocretin-1 does not cross the blood–brain barrier. In animal models, it has been observed that intraventricular administration of ORX suppressed narcolepsy symptoms in mice subjected to ORX/ataxin-3 neuronal ablation. Intrathecal ORX administration via an implantable pump was also proposed as a therapy for refractory patients with NT1. Unfortunately, these models have not been developed in humans, so the development of peptide analogues of hypocretin that cross the blood–brain barrier and act centrally via non-invasive routes of administration would be the most viable future therapy. On the other hand, a non-invasive method through intranasal administration of ORX, directing the drugs to the brain along the olfactory and trigeminal neural pathways, could also be of interest as it has been shown to decrease the amount of REM sleep and REM sleep is more stable, but no effect has been observedin regard to drowsiness. At present, intranasal hypocretin is not a viable treatment [10, 11].

C. Transformation of stem cells into orexin neurons: in rats, patches have been transplanted with posterior hypothalamus cells causing a reduction in drowsiness. Hypothalamic neurons have been generated in vitro from embryonic stem cells and pluripotent stem cells. This therapy could therefore become a final option for very severe and drug-resistant narcoleptic patients.

D. Orexin-based gene therapy: the use of recombinant viruses has been postulated. Studies have been promising (improving symptoms in narcoleptics). More studies are needed to establish the safety and efficacy of the technique, but they could be future therapies.

E. Immune therapy: as mentioned above, by the time a patient is symptomatic, ORX neurons may already be irreversibly destroyed. A recent article used a highly sensitive method to detect rare T cell populations and found the presence of CD4+ T cells that recognised prepro-ORX peptide epitopes in NT1 and that have not been observed in healthy controls. Based on the model of immune-mediated hypocretinergic neurone destruction, immunotherapy applied at the onset of the disease to prevent neuronal death was postulated as a treatment. To date, several studies have been conducted implementing this methodology in narcoleptics, but the existing data are based on a very small number of patients, and they are uncontrolled case studies. Some of the different therapeutic strategies that have been tried include: corticosteroids, intravenous immunoglobulins (IVIG), plasmapheresis, rituximab, etc. with variable efficacy, possibly due to the lack of safety if the treatment was applied at the onset of the disease and not when the situation was already irreversible. A study has been published of a patient who received treatment with IVIG for 15 days right at the onset of the disease, completely reversing the clinical symptoms (EDS and cataplexy) and normalising the levels of ORX in CSF, which were initially undetectable. Regarding new immune-based therapies. A recent review has been published, presenting several treatments targeting NT1, including: Natalizumab, Fingolimod, Abatacept, monoclonal antibodies targeting T or B cells, TNF alpha inhibitors, Anakinra, antigen-specific therapies or Cyclophosphamide. In another study they propose that for future trials with immunotherapy, patients should have a specific profile with clear selection criteria, benefiting above all, those with ongoing inflammatory or autoimmune processes [12].

5. Conclusion

Recent years have seen a resurgence of new lines of therapy for the treatment of narcolepsy. These new future prospects predict a promising prognosis in terms of being able to guarantee a better quality of life for patients with narcolepsy, perhaps even a possible correction of the hypocretin deficit, completely resolving the symptomatology and achieving complete control of the disease. Future lines of research should be based on the discovery of new reliable biomarkers to be able to identify the patients who best respond to immunomodulators and, of course, on the discovery of the underlying mechanisms related to the destruction of hypocretin-producing neurons. On the other hand, we have highlighted the lack of clinical trials in some specific groups, such as pregnant women or the elderly population. In addition, further trials in patients with common comorbidities such as psychiatric disorders or cardiovascular risk factors would be of interest.

Conflict of interest

The authors declare that they have no conflicts of interest.

Author details

Juan José Ortega-Albás*, Raquel López García, Alfonso Martínez Martínez, Sonia Carratalá Monfort, Juan Antonio Royo Prats, Laura Albiol Varela and Patricia Ortega Gabás
Sleep Unit, General Universitary Hospital of Castellón, Castellón de la Plana, España

*Address all correspondence to: jjoralbas@gmail.com

References

[1] Bassetti C, Adamantidis A, Burdakov D, Han F, Gay S, et al. Narcolepsy: Clinical spectrum, aetiopathophysiology, diagnosis and treatment. Nature Reviews. Neurology. 2019;**15**(9):519-539. DOI: 10.1038/s41582-019-0226-9

[2] Reading PJ. Update on narcolepsy. Journal of Neurology. 2019;**266**: 1809-1815. DOI: 10.1007/s00415-019-09310-3

[3] Scammell TE. Narcolepsy. The New England Journal of Medicine. 2015;**373**: 2654-2662. DOI: 10.1056/NEJMra1500587

[4] Golden EC, Lipford MC. Narcolepsy: Diagnosis and management. Cleveland Clinic Journal of Medicine. 2018;**85**(12): 959-959

[5] Abad VC, Guilleminault C. New developments in the management of narcolepsy. Nature and Science of Sleep. 2017;**9**:39-57. DOI: 10.2147/NSS.S103467

[6] Dauvilliers Y, Bassetti C, Lammers GJ, Arnulf I, Mayer G, Rodenbeck A, et al. Pitolisant versus placebo or modafinil in patients with narcolepsy: A double-blind, randomised trial. Lancet Neurology. 2013;**12**(11):1068-1075. DOI: 10.1016/S1474-4422(13)70225-4

[7] Powell J, Piszczatoski C, Garland S. Solriamfetol for excessive sleepiness in narcolepsy and obstructive sleep apnea. The Annals of Pharmacotherapy. 2020; **54**(10):1016-1020. DOI: 10.1177/1060028020915537

[8] Bassetti CLA, Kallweit U, Vignatelli L, Plazzi G, Lecendreu M, et al. European guideline and expert statements on the management of narcolepsy in adults and children. Journal of Sleep Research. 2021;**25**: e13387. DOI: 10.1111/jsr13387

[9] Thorpy MJ. Recently approved and upcoming treatments for narcolepsy. CNS Drugs. 2020;**34**:9-27. DOI: 10.1007/s40263-019-00689-1

[10] Arias-Carrión O, Murillo Rodriguez E. Effects of hypocretin/orexin cell transplantation on narcoleptic-like sleep behavior in rats. PLoS One. 2014;**9**(4): e95342. DOI: 10.1371/journal.pone.0095342

[11] Pérez Carbonell L. Treatment of excessive daytime sleepiness in patients with narcolepsy. Current Treatment Options in Neurology. 2019;**21**(11):57. DOI: 10.1007/s11940-019-0595-9

[12] Barateau L, Dauvilliers Y. Recent advances in treatment for narcolepsy. Therapeutic Advances in Neurological Disorders. 2019;**12**:1756286419875622. DOI: 10.1177/1756286419875622

Chapter 4

The Pharmacology of Parasomnias and Movement Disorders of Sleep

Gregory S. Carter

Abstract

The treatment of parasomnias and sleep related movement disorders is not always pharmacologic, indeed, some of these disorders respond to behavioral approaches without the risks of pharmaceuticals. This chapter endeavors to pull forward the disorders in which pharmacologic treatment is the best choice and lay out the pharmacologic properties of the treatments. It is not the goal of this chapter to present an encyclopedic review of the parasomnias and sleep related movement disorders. It is, however, the intent of this chapter to comprehensively review pharmacologic treatments used in the management of the disorders in which drug use is most necessary. The pharmacokinetic and pharmacodynamic properties and known risks of these pharmaceuticals are presented and discussed. When more than one pharmaceutical is used clinically within a class of drugs, thorough review of selected drugs is presented. The chapter includes investigations, mostly human studies, of the drugs discussed. The author's extensive experience in pharmacology, neurology, and sleep medicine take the chapter through pharmacological information a clinician needs to guide the management of these disorders.

Keywords: Treatment of parasomnias, movement disorders of sleep, pharmacology of sleep disorders, comparison of the benzodiazepines, comparison of the dopamine receptor agonists, gabapentin and pregabalin for sleep disorders, risks of sleep medications, melatonin, restless leg syndrome, alcohol, caffeine, and opiate effects on sleep disorders

1. Introduction

Henri Roger first gave us the term "parasomnia" in 1932 [1]. Subsequently, parasomnias have been extensively described and classified into non-REM-related parasomnias and REM-related parasomnias, so designated for the sleep stage from which the parasomnia emerges [2]. Though there is overlap in treatment options for the parasomnias, treatment most often follows semiology and pathophysiology. Sleep-related movement disorders are likewise varied in their presentations [3]. The treatment of parasomnias and sleep-related movement disorders relies on removal or avoidance of precipitants, behavioral techniques, prosthetic or dental devices, as well as, medications. Multi-pronged approaches including behavioral techniques in addition to medications may be most effective. The use of medication is still a necessary component of care in illnesses with significant immediate and long-term complications. This includes serious complications to the individual suffering from these sleep disorders, as well as, their bed partners and others within their circle of family and friends. In the body of this chapter, I will review the parasomnias and sleep-related

IntechOpen

movement disorders with behavioral and pharmaceutical approaches to treatment. Where behavioral approaches alone are much preferred, this chapter will not delve into the physiology, psychology or known pathology of the disorder. Where pharmaceutical approaches are common, the chapter will briefly discuss the pathophysiology of the disorder and the desirable treatment strategies from clinical studies and expert opinion. Drug classes will be fully addressed in individual sections. These sections will discuss the pharmacokinetics, pharmacodynamics, and adverse effect profiles of the more commonly prescribed drugs within these classes, comparing them by popularity, desirable properties, and risks of adverse events. Lastly, in the conclusion this chapter will briefly review the current controversies of pharmacologic treatment.

2. The parasomnias

The parasomnias can be divided into the non-REM parasomnias, the REM parasomnias, the overlap parasomnias, and others which defy definition by sleep stage [4]. To best understand these differences, it is necessary to have some knowledge of role sleep plays in normal physiology. The sleep stages show a cyclic pattern of light sleep (N1) proceeding to common sleep (N2), then to slow wave or deep sleep (N3) and finally rapid eye movement (REM) sleep. The cycles gradually change with more N3 sleep in the first half of the night and more REM sleep in the second half of the night. These sleep cycles have been shown to serve multiple physiologic and homeostatic functions, but for the purposes of this chapter, deep sleep (N3) has been associated with the arousal disorders (confusional arousals, sleep walking, and sleep terrors) and REM sleep has been associated with dream enactment or REM sleep behavior disorders and nightmares. Each of these disorders demand therapeutic approaches that may not work for the others, i.e., sedation may be helpful (at least temporarily) for REM sleep parasomnias, but be counter-productive in the arousal disorders.

2.1 Clinical evaluation

The clinical differentiation of the parasomnias demands a careful and complete history and physical exam. Witnesses to and video recordings of the parasomnia are invaluable. Precipitants for parasomnias include sleep-related breathing disorders, sleep deprivation and insufficient sleep for age, emotional trauma and chronic mental illness, narcolepsy, endocrine disorders including hypothyroidism, diabetes, and perimenstrual distress, degenerative brain disorders, such as Parkinsonism and dementia with Lewy bodies, head injury and stroke, epileptic and non-epileptic seizures, and medications including lithium, neuroleptics, anticholinergics, antidepressants, sedative-hypnotics, opioids, and various recreational drugs including alcohol. Very high dose caffeine consumption is another concern as is current marijuana use and the use of illegal drugs such as fentanyl and cocaine. A family history of parasomnia may or may not be present on initial evaluation. A thorough physical examination may reveal findings consistent with sleep apnea or respiratory compromise, thyroid enlargement or tenderness, neurologic deficits or psychiatric abnormalities. Given the spectrum of parasomnias and varying etiologies underlying them, if the clinician's assessment misses an important precipitant or co-morbidity, pharmacologic management will likely fail or cause adverse effects.

2.2 Arousal disorders

The arousal disorders arise out of deep sleep (N3) and are felt to represent parasomnias emerging from difficulty completely awaking from sleep.

A.	Recurrent episodes of incomplete awakening from sleep
B.	Inappropriate or absent responsiveness to efforts of others to intervene or redirect the person during the episode
C.	Limited (e.g., a single visual scene) or no associated cognition or dream imagery
D.	Partial or complete amnesia for the episode
E.	The disturbance is not better explained by another sleep disorder, mental disorder, medical condition, medication or substance use

Notes
The events usually occur during the first third of the major sleep episode
The individual may continue to appear confused and disoriented for several minutes or longer following the episode.

Table 1.
General diagnostic criteria for disorders of arousal (criteria A-E must be met) [2].

These disorders consist predominantly of confusional arousals, sleep walking and sleep terrors and effect children under 11 years of age more than adults. There is a wide variance in reports of prevalence of arousal disorders from 9–45% of children [2, 4–7]. The lifetime prevalence in individuals over 15 years of age falls to 2.9% to 4.2%. The diagnostic criteria are presented in **Table 1**. Genetic factors [8], infections, sleep deprivation, and obstructive sleep apnea [9] can all be predisposing factors, whose elimination may prevent recurrent events. With the exception of epilepsy, pharmacotherapy may not be effective and may actually worsen symptoms [10]. Reassurance and behavioral approaches such as creating a safe sleeping environment, anticipatory or scheduled awakenings, cognitive behavioral therapy [10, 11], and hypnosis [12] are among the non-pharmacologic options.

Use of drugs in the developing brain is a concern for pharmacologists due to the extreme plasticity of immature neuronal networks. Another concern for the use of pharmaceutical agents in children is the tendency of the disorders to resolve spontaneously as a child matures. Proserpio et al. [13] laid out four indications for initiation of pharmacotherapy. The first is persistence of frequent episodes despite elimination of predisposing factors. The second is high risk of injury. The third is significant functional impairment, and the fourth is potential legal consequences. In the presence of 2–4, there may not be time to pursue behavioral approaches to management.

The most frequently used drugs for arousal disorders are the benzodiazepines. Antidepressant drugs have been used less frequently. Of note, none of these drugs has an FDA indication for their use in arousal disorders or have any large-scale controlled studies of their efficacy. The very long-acting benzodiazepine, clonazepam, has been the most frequently used agent [14–16] though other benzodiazepines including alprazolam and diazepam have been used in adult sleep terrors and sleepwalking. Antidepressant drugs including sertraline, paroxetine [17], clomipramine, imipramine [18], and trazodone [19] have been used in small case series. Case reports have also shown efficacy in the treatment of arousal disorders for melatonin [20, 21], hydroxytryptophan [22, 23], and ramelteon [24].

2.2.1 Sleep-related Hypermotor epilepsy

Nocturnal frontal lobe epilepsy, otherwise known as sleep-related hypermotor epilepsy, can present as recurrent, intractable confusional arousals [25, 26]. Routine polysomnography is not as helpful in differentiating an arousal disorder from sleep-related hypermotor epilepsy as is video-electroencephalographic recording in an inpatient epilepsy monitoring center. While this is an expensive evaluation option, home video recording via cell phone camera, stereotypical behavior of the events, frequency up to nightly, persistence into adulthood, and the presence of a brain disorder can guide a clinician's decision to proceed [27]. In the author's experience in a busy university sleep clinic, less than 5% of adult patients presenting with arousal disorders are referred for epilepsy monitoring, however, 30% of the patients who were referred for epilepsy monitoring were diagnosed with likely or definite sleep-related hypermotor epilepsy. As a side note, treatment trials with anti-seizure drugs in these patients are not helpful for differentiation, as the pharmacologic control of sleep-related hypermotor epilepsy is often challenging.

2.3 REM parasomnias

The REM sleep related parasomnias most prominently include REM sleep behavior disorder and nightmare disorder [2]. REM sleep behavior disorder is often managed with medications, but nightmare disorder is more often treated with behavioral interventions. The prevalence of REM sleep behavioral disorder (REMSBD) is unknown but has been estimated to be 0.38% of the general population, increasing in frequency with age [28, 29]. It is more prevalent in men and usually emerges after age 50 [2]. There is a prominent association in older patients with the synucleinopathies [30]. The differential in younger patients can be quite wide. This parasomnia can be co-morbid with narcolepsy, brain tumors, antidepressant medications, and neurodevelopmental disorders [2]. Severe obstructive sleep apnea can cause dream enactment that mirrors REM sleep behavior disorder [31]. A variety of medications have been implicated in the precipitation of REM sleep behavior disorder. Antidepressants including venlafaxine, mirtazapine, and selective serotonin reuptake inhibitors, but not the dopamine reuptake inhibitor bupropion [32], can precipitate REMSBD. Medications including beta-blockers, anticholinesterase inhibitors, and selegiline have been reported to precipitate REMSBD [2]. Nightmares may occur in 60–75% of children; however, frequent nightmares are far less common occurring in only 1–5% of children [33]. Post-traumatic stress disorder is a common cause of nightmares in adults [34], but 2–8% of the general population may have troublesome nightmares. Various pharmaceuticals can precipitate nightmares. These include drugs affecting the neurotransmission of norepinephrine, serotonin, and dopamine such as antidepressants, antihypertensives, and dopamine receptor agonists. In addition, the withdrawal of a REM sleep suppressant can precipitate the complaint of nightmares. Varenicline, a nicotinic antagonist, may commonly induce nightmares [35]. The clinical management of nightmares includes removing as many predisposing factors as possible.

The chapter will not discuss parasomnias, such as exploding head syndrome and sleep related hallucinations, that are treated with reassurance and very rarely with drugs. Sleep enuresis may occur in 15–20% of five-year-old's [2]. It is more common in boys. Non-pharmacologic treatments are superior when the etiology is obstructive sleep apnea [36], ingestion of high doses of caffeine or psychosocial stressors. Nightly desmopressin is used when indicated for frequent intractable sleep enuresis. Pharmacologic management is necessary for urinary tract infections, diabetes insipidus, diabetes mellitus, or nocturnal epilepsy [2]. Fortunately, improvement occurs with age in these children.

3. Sleep related movement disorders

The sleep related movement disorders consist of restless leg syndrome, periodic limb movement disorder, sleep related leg cramps, sleep related bruxism, the sleep related rhythmic movement disorders, sleep related myoclonus at sleep onset, propriospinal myoclonus at sleep onset [2]. Benign sleep myoclonus of infancy is different in that more than half of these infants have neonatal opioid withdrawal syndrome [37]. Sleep related rhythmic movement disorders, sleep related myoclonus at sleep onset, and propriospinal myoclonus at sleep onset, and benign sleep myoclonus of infancy are very rarely treated with pharmaceuticals once the diagnosis is made. Reassurance and building a safe bedroom environment are the treatments of choice. Likewise, sleep related bruxism (SRB) is best treated with oral devices that protect the teeth. Sleep related bruxism has its highest incidence in childhood, occurring in 14–17% of children before decreasing over the life span to 3% of older persons [38]. Sleep related breathing disorders are often co-morbid with sleep bruxism [39] though the relationship is unclear. More recently, botulinum toxin has been used for intractable sleep bruxism [40, 41]. Sleep related leg cramps are common. Almost all adults have had a leg cramp during sleep, and likely during wakefulness. Nightly leg cramps are reported in 6% of adults older than 60 [42]. The precipitants of sleep related leg cramps are as numerous as the over-the-counter dietary supplements used to treat them. The fact that no supplement has dominated the market speaks to their success. Predisposing factors include, but are not limited to, hypokalemia, hypocalcemia, hypomagnesemia, vigorous exercise, prolonged standing, oral contraceptives, diuretics, and long duration of action beta blockers [43]. Prescription medications including carisoprodol, diltiazem, gabapentin, orphenadrine, verapamil, have been used with success that likely does not significantly exceed placebo, presuming there were any controlled trials.

3.1 Periodic limb movement disorder/restless leg syndrome

The remaining sleep related movement disorders are the closely related periodic limb movement disorder and restless leg syndrome. Restless leg syndrome (RLS) is a clinical symptom complex. Periodic limb movements (PLM) are a polysomnographic finding seen very frequently with the symptom complex of restless leg syndrome. When the symptom complex of restless leg syndrome is absent, the polysomnographic finding of periodic limb movements become a disorder when there is clinically significant sleep disturbance or impairment in mental, physical, social, occupational, educational, behavioral, or other areas of functioning [2]. Periodic limb movements are seen on polysomnograms with greater frequency as patients grow older, though not all of these patients complain of sleep disturbance or nonrestorative sleep. Patients with periodic limb movement disorder can develop symptom worsening with prescription drugs including selective serotonin reuptake inhibitors, tricyclic antidepressants, lithium, and dopamine receptor antagonists. Low brain iron levels as manifested in peripheral blood by low ferritin levels and low total iron binding percentage are another precipitant. As with RLS, gene variants have been identified accounting for a fraction of affected individuals with a family history [3]. Care must be taken on polysomnograms to separate arousals secondary to limb movements from arousals due to sleep related breathing disorders. Distinction of periodic limb movements of sleep with no secondary sleep arousal versus periodic limb movement disorder with secondary arousal can be difficult. This is especially true of patients undergoing polysomnograms for another sleep pathology, such as suspected sleep related breathing disorder. The use of PLM associated cortical electroencephalographic arousals to determine clinical significance of periodic limb movements may thus be misleading. Cortical arousals as measured by an abrupt change to 3 seconds of 8 cycles per second rhythms (or higher frequencies) within 0.5 second of the limb movement [44] may be more subjective than the rule would suggest. Thus, the decision to treat or not to treat a patient with a periodic limb movement index of greater than 15 limb movements per hour can be dependent on the treating physician's overall clinical assessment. Restless leg syndrome is an urge to move the legs usually accompanied by an uncomfortable sensation in the legs. The need to move worsens with rest, is relieved by movement, and emerges in a drug naïve patient at a specific time in their circadian cycle, usually in the evening [2]. Between 21 and 57% of patients will have arm symptoms. Sleep initiation and maintenance may be quite difficult for these patients resulting in their seeking medical care. The overall prevalence of RLS is estimated to be 5–10% in Europe and the United States but lower in Asia. Both prevalence and severity increase with age. Family history (obtained in 40–92% of cases) and the female gender confer increased risk. Pregnancy, especially the third trimester, has a risk three times greater risk than the general population. Restless leg syndrome is a clinical diagnosis that requires differentiation from the pain of leg cramps, arthralgias, myalgias, neuropathic pain, neuroleptic-induced akathisia, subtle spasticity from myelopathy, and anxiety-induced restlessness and repetitive movements. Many of these patients require prescription medications for control of symptoms. Medications for RLS and PLM disorder fall into four classes which will be discussed in depth later in this chapter. The four classes are the dopamine agonists, the alpha 2 delta subunit neuronal voltage-gated calcium channel blockers, the benzodiazepines and the opioids.

4. Implications for pharmacological management

The prescription drugs used in parasomnias and sleep related movement disorders fall into several classes. The benzodiazepines are broadly used for parasomnias and sleep related movement disorders. Melatonin is also widely used for parasomnias. Antidepressants with various pharmacodynamic properties are often used both to suppress parasomnias and treat comorbid mood disorders. Prazosin is a drug that has been widely used for nightmares. The dopamine receptor agonists are used with great frequency for both periodic limb movements and restless legs syndrome. The alpha 2 delta subunit neuronal voltage-gated calcium channel blockers are used predominantly for RLS/PLMD and other disorders. The final class of prescription drugs is the opioids.

We cannot go further into this chapter without taking into consideration the ideal properties of a drug to treat sleep disorders. These properties of oral medications include good gastro-duodenal absorption, ability to cross the blood brain barrier, a metabolic rate and duration of action that match the need for intervention, and a low potential for drug interactions. Low short-term and long-term effects on the molecular receptor target are also important. Direct and indirect adverse effects are additional determinants of patient compliance and satisfaction.

5. The Benzodiazapines

The benzodiazepines were first synthesized by Leo Sternbach in 1955 [45]. The benzodiazepines had activity on the neuronal chloride ionophore augmenting the effect of gamma aminobutyric acid (GABA) in facilitating sleep, sedation, anti-anxiety effects, and muscle relaxation. Hundreds of benzodiazepines were synthesized between 1960 and 1980 [46], but only a few have had commercial success. With the marketing of chlordiazepoxide in 1960 and diazepam in 1963 the benzodiazepines increased rapidly in prescription frequency [47]. The utility of these drugs as anti-anxiety agents and sedative hypnotics was important to this rise, but safety characteristics were equally important. The therapeutic window of the benzodiazepines was much wider than the barbiturates and the lethal dose for 50% of animals in toxicology studies of diazepam was ten times that of secobarbital [48]. Over 50 years the growth of benzodiazepine prescribing was substantial. In 2017 there were 45.0 million alprazolam, 26.4 million lorazepam, 29.2 million clonazepam, 12.6 million diazepam, and 7.0 million temazepam prescriptions dispensed in the United States [49]. The benzodiazepines were placed in Schedule IV of the Controlled Substances Act of 1971. Alprazolam was one of the top three prescription drugs diverted to the illicit market. While the benzodiazepines were less dangerous than barbiturates due to a wider therapeutic window, there were still 14 deaths associated with benzodiazepines in 2017, most due to intentional overdose. According to the National Institute on Drug Abuse there were a total of 70,630 overdose deaths in the United States in 2019 [50]. Most of those deaths were due to opioids, mainly fentanyl. The benzodiazepines were involved in 9,711 of those deaths, usually in combination with opioids. By comparison there were 5,175 deaths in 2019 associated with antidepressants. Many dose-related adverse effects of benzodiazepines resulted from depression of the central nervous system including drowsiness, impaired judgment, diminished motor skills, and anterograde amnesia, causing falls and confusion in the elderly, breathing problems in symptomatic sleep apnea or chronic pulmonary disease, driving impairment, and worsened job performance.

5.1 Pharmacokinetics and pharmacodynamics

The GABA system is the location of the primary pharmacodynamics of the benzodiazepines [51]. This system is the major inhibitory system in the central nervous system, thus the drug effect producing central nervous system depression. The GABA-A receptors upon which the benzodiazepines produce their effect are pentameric ligand-gated chloride ion channels. There are 21 different subunit isoforms within the GABA-A chloride ionophore. These are divided into eight families which within their family share 70% of their amino acid sequences. These subunit families are classified into alpha, beta, gamma, delta, epsilon, pi, omega, and rho. The first four of these are most important for benzodiazepine action. The structure most frequently seen in the brain consists of two alpha subunits and two beta subunits and one gamma or, less frequently, one delta subunit [52]. The neurotransmitter GABA binds to the interface between the alpha and beta subunits to open the chloride ionophore. Benzodiazepines bind to the interface of the alpha and gamma subunits. The benzodiazepine binding produces an allosteric change making the GABA receptor more sensitive, producing benzodiazepine clinical effects. Of interest for future drug development, the alpha subunit family contains alpha-1 through alpha-6 subunits which vary in benzodiazepine sensitivities and specific clinical effects [53, 54]. Thus, alpha subunit composition containing alpha-1 is associated with sedation, amnesia, anti-seizure activity, and addiction propensity. Alpha-2 subunits are associated with anti-anxiety propensity, muscle relaxation, cognitive disturbance, and analgesic properties. Alpha-5 subunits are associated with learning, memory, and muscle relaxation.

While the basic 3 ring skeletal molecular structure of the benzodiazepines is the same, different additions to this molecular structure yield important differences in properties. Classification of these additions to the basic benzodiazepine nucleus use 7 groupings, five of which are important to this discussion. The triazolo group (alprazolam, triazolam, estazolam) and the imidazo group (midazolam) include drugs that are closely related structurally. Likewise, the 3-hydroxy group (lorazepam, oxazepam, and temazepam) all have similar molecular structures. The

2-keto group, including diazepam and the 7-nitro group including clonazepam are significantly different structurally from the other benzodiazepines. These molecular structure differences contribute to the pharmacologic properties of these drugs. The GABA-A receptors also change in response to exogenous factors including benzodiazepine exposure. Internalization of the receptor complex leads to degradation and altered composition of the pentameric structure, rendering the receptor complex less sensitive and less numerous.

There are two prime factors in the choice of a benzodiazepine, half-life and potency. A low potency and long half-life benzodiazepine is diazepam and a low potency and short half-life benzodiazepine is temazepam. A high potency and long half-life benzodiazepine is clonazepam and two high potency short half-life benzodiazepines are alprazolam and lorazepam. The pharmacodynamic effects of the benzodiazepines are similar. Thus, pharmacokinetic properties, potency, dosing requirements, and efficacy have determined usage. Several of the benzodiazepines have been used in the pharmacologic treatment of parasomnias and sleep related movement disorders, and as a class may be the most frequent and widely used pharmacological management. Four commonly used agents are described below in alphabetical order.

5.2 Alprazolam

This triazolo benzodiazepine was approved by the FDA in 1981 for the treatment of panic disorder. The doses of alprazolam for panic disorder were very high, up to 6–12 mg per day. It quickly became the most widely prescribed benzodiazepine shortly after marketing. The oral absorption of alprazolam after a single 1 mg dose is rapid with an oral bioavailability of 80–100% and peak plasma concentrations in young males occurring within 0.7 to 1.8 hours after administration [55]. It is a CYP3A4 substrate subject to multiple metabolic inducers and inhibitors. The metabolic products of hepatic microsomal oxidation yield alpha-hydroxy and 4-hydroxy alprazolam which have 10% of the plasma concentrations of the parent drug and lower affinity for benzodiazepine receptors. A number of drugs may impair metabolism of alprazolam, including fluoxetine [56] and propoxyphene, enhancing central nervous system effects. The elimination half-life in young men ranged from 9 to 16 hours. Healthy elderly men had significantly longer half-lives with a mean of 19 hours versus a mean of 11 hours in young men [57].

Alprazolam falls into the intermediate range among benzodiazepines in regards to lipid solubility (50% of diazepam). This characteristic determines the degree of uptake into the brain [58] as well as the speed at which alprazolam enters the brain. Several studies have demonstrated that the steady state plasma concentrations of alprazolam after multiple dosing are proportional to the daily dose and do not change the half-life [59–61].

The general binding characteristics are similar to the other benzodiazepines, however, the receptor affinity of alprazolam (K_i) of 3.4 nm is tighter than diazepam's K_i of 5.3 nm [62]. This reflects the potency enhancement from the chloride at position 8 on the phenyl ring along with the triazolo ring. This enhancement is even tighter for another triazolobenzodiazepine, triazolam, with its remarkable receptor affinity (K_i) of 0.5 nm [63]. A unique characteristic not shared by other benzodiazepines [62] was seen with low doses (0.02–0.05 mg/kg) of alprazolam in mice [64]. An increased benzodiazepine receptor number was seen compared to the decreased receptor number seen with other benzodiazepines and high dose alprazolam.

Clinical information regarding the use of alprazolam in REM sleep behavioral disorder is limited [65]. Published results [66, 67] yield varying utility, though this author's results [68, 69] have been quite positive at doses of alprazolam 0.5 mg at bedtime. Alprazolam would appear to have good pharmacokinetic and pharmacodynamic properties for use in nocturnal parasomnias when a benzodiazepine is indicated. Currently, however, it is not frequently prescribed for that purpose. Of note, in the elderly (>65 years old) there is a significant and dramatic dose related increase in sedation and neuromotor testing decrement between alprazolam doses of 0.5 mg and 2.0 mg [60].

5.3 Clonazepam

Clonazepam is the most common drug used for parasomnias. It is limited to oral administration, but has been used widely for panic disorder and psychosis, as well as, having anti-seizure properties shared with diazepam, lorazepam, and clobazam. This 7-nitro group benzodiazepine differs structurally from other benzodiazepines resulting in high potency and tight binding affinity (Ki 2.0 nm) to benzodiazepine receptors. Clonazepam is rapidly and completely absorbed after oral administration and reaches peak plasma concentrations in 1–4 hours [70]. Absolute bioavailability is 90%. It is highly metabolized by the hepatic microsomal system with less than 2% being excreted unchanged in the urine. The remarkable property of this drug is its long half-life of 30–40 hours. The constant presence of the drug with multiple dosing results in benzodiazepine downregulation with loss of both high affinity binding and receptor number [71, 72]. Specific clonazepam binding was reduced by 24.9% with chronic administration. This likely explains the loss of efficacy and development of tolerance with multiple dosing. Clonazepam, more than lorazepam or alprazolam, produced impairment on neuromotor tasks [73, 74]. Alprazolam showed significantly faster recovery on testing performance than either clonazepam or lorazepam even though lorazepam has a similar half-life. Ellinwood et al. also found that the equivalent dose of alprazolam was half the dosage level of the other two drugs, a phenomenon that could not be explained by receptor affinity. The length of impairment with lorazepam was greater than clonazepam presumably secondary to its greater lipid solubility.

Clonazepam is currently the suggested treatment for REM sleep behavioral disorder with more published studies than other drugs that have been used in this disorder [65]. Clonazepam showed efficacy in 80% of 200 patients at the Minnesota Regional Sleep Disorders Center [66, 67]. There is concern, however, for the use of clonazepam in dementia, gait disorders, and obstructive sleep apnea due to reports of worsening of each of these with chronic clonazepam dosing. Aurora et al. [65] reviewed the adverse event profile of clonazepam and found reports of sedation, impotence, early morning loss of motor coordination, confusion, and memory dysfunction.

5.4 Diazepam

Diazepam, within six years of it being marketed, became the most prescribed drug in the United States from 1969 to 1982 [49]. Diazepam has chemical properties of lipid solubility and non-ionization at physiological pH that made absorption through the gut wall and cerebral capillaries rapid, allowing potent brain concentrations within minutes. Peak blood levels with oral dosing are achieved in 1–2 hours. The half-life varies between 20 and 80 hours making the drug a long-acting agent. Diazepam gained multiple uses including anti-anxiety, sedative, anti-seizure, anti-vertigo, and muscle relaxant effects due to its action on both central and peripheral benzodiazepine receptors. It is available in oral, rectal, and parenteral formulations. Hepatic metabolism of diazepam produces an active metabolite, desmethyldiazepam (DMD), which at steady state with repeated dosing eventually has a higher plasma concentration than its parent drug. The elimination of DMD occurs much more slowly than diazepam with a half-life of 36–96 hours. If diazepam is discontinued, withdrawal symptoms can occur ranging from anxiety to seizures with higher doses. Diazepam remains a secondary benzodiazepine for both non-REM and REM sleep related parasomnias. It is a tertiary treatment when first and second-line treatments have failed.

5.5 Lorazepam

Lorazepam has many uses in addition to its indication for anxiety with depression. It has been used as a hypnotic and as a treatment for panic disorder, alcoholic delirium tremens, status epilepticus, and pre-procedural sedation [73]. It is available in oral and parenteral formulations. Its use for parasomnias and sleep-related movement disorders has been limited and Aurora et al. [65] did not report lorazepam being used for REM sleep behavior disorder.

Lorazepam is one of the 3-hydroxy group of benzodiazepines. This drug is available in oral and parenteral formulations and is metabolized by glucuronidation thus the absence of concern for hepatic impairment or an active metabolite. It has utility for anti- anxiety and anti-seizure applications. It is absorbed quickly after oral administration with a time to peak plasma levels of 1–5 hours [70]. Like diazepam, lorazepam is highly lipophilic and quickly crosses the blood–brain barrier. It is rapidly absorbed when administered orally and has a half-life of 10–20 hours. As discussed in Section 4.1b, lorazepam has a longer duration of action than might be expected for its elimination half-life. The ortho chloride on the ring structures of lorazepam, clonazepam, and triazolam increase receptor binding and thus potency. The tighter binding may be the reason for the longer duration of action [73].

6. Melatonin

Endogenous melatonin is a hormone secreted by the pineal gland in tandem with the circadian rhythm. Studies of melatonin revealed sedative properties leading to its use in sleep disorders [75–77]. Melatonin is considered a dietary supplement by the Food and Drug Administration in the United States and thus the formulations are not subject to the regulations that govern prescription medications mentioned in this chapter.

Buscemi et al. [78] did a clinical review of 14 randomized controlled trials of exogenous melatonin for sleep disorders. The meta-analysis showed a reduced sleep latency of 11.7 minutes (CI: −18.2, −5.2), but this was most significant in those patients with delayed sleep-phase syndrome. All of the patients studied carried diagnoses of either insomnia or delayed sleep-phase disorder. No doses higher than 5 mg per night were used and half the studies used no more than 3 mg per night. Of the 222 combined participants, 13 reported headaches, 10 dizziness, 3 nausea, and 3 drowsiness. In all of these there was no significant difference between melatonin and placebo.

Moroni et al. [79] conducted another systematic review looking at 19 published studies utilizing different formulations of exogenous melatonin. Most of the studies reviewed used low dose melatonin (<5 mg). The immediate-release formulations produced a decrease in sleep onset latency and the sustained release formulations had a greater effect on reducing wakefulness after sleep onset. Oral formulations of melatonin had variability in both absorption and metabolism. There were no adverse effects noted in very short-term therapy among healthy research participants.

The amount of melatonin that enters the systemic circulation is decreased by first-pass metabolism. The hepatic enzyme involved in metabolism of melatonin is CYP1A2 [80, 81]. This enzyme has higher activity in males, likely contributing to the gender differences seen in one study [82] which showed almost three times higher systemic circulation concentrations in females. An older group of research participants also showed three times the maximal concentration in their systemic circulation [83].

The Standards of Practice Committee of the American Academy of Sleep Medicine (AASM) published recommendations which included a suggestion that melatonin be used for the treatment of REM sleep behavior disorder [65]. They noted that melatonin had been shown to be effective with few adverse effects. There are actually only a few reports showing efficacy of melatonin in parasomnias [75, 84]. This author's experience in a large university sleep clinic confirms the efficacy of melatonin in some patients, but the patients with parasomnias treated successfully with melatonin comprise less than half of the patients treated successfully with benzodiazepines [68].

Dose related adverse effects were reported including headache, morning sleepiness, and delusions/hallucinations [75]. In another set of AASM recommendations for the management of circadian disorders [85] melatonin adverse effects were discussed in greater depth. There were no serious adverse effects, however, headaches, somnolence, hypotension, hypertension, gastrointestinal upset, and exacerbation of alopecia areata were all reported. An increase in depressive symptoms [86], impairment of glucose tolerance [87], and reproductive function [88] were reported. Studies beyond 3 months of melatonin use and studies in pediatrics were and remain scarce. Pediatric concerns were reported including potential effects on growth hormone regulation with high dose melatonin (10 mg) [89]. There was additional thought that the efficacy in pediatric parasomnias might be related to an indirect effect of improving sleep rather than a direct effect of melatonin [65].

In conclusion, melatonin is efficacious in some patients with REM sleep behavioral disorder and possibly other parasomnias with no serious adverse effects.

7. The antidepressants

There have been many antidepressants used in patients with a variety of parasomnias either as primary or concomitant therapy. Parasomnias can be co-morbid with mental health disorders leading to antidepressant treatment. The confounding factor is that some parasomnias and sleep-related movement disorders may be exacerbated or even elicited by antidepressant therapy [90–94]. Lam et al. [95] used a questionnaire to identify patients with parasomnias then confirmed the diagnosis via a clinical interview. Of the 1235 participants who completed the interview 22.3% had clinically confirmed somnambulism, sleep-related eating disorder, or sleep related injury. REM sleep behavior disorder (RSBD) was the cause of sleep related injury in 66.7% of the subgroup of participants with sleep related injury. The use of selective serotonin reuptake inhibitors (SSRIs) was associated with symptoms of RSBD in 5% of participants. Of the 29 participants diagnosed with somnambulism 34.5% were using sedating antidepressants [96].

Drug-induced RSBD has been further associated with the tricyclic antidepressant clomipramine and the monoamine oxidase inhibitors selegiline and phenelzine [94]. In spite of these risks co-morbid psychiatric disorders often lead to treatment with antidepressants in individuals with parasomnias. There are also a variety of case reports of the effective use of antidepressants for management of parasomnias. Imipramine was used successfully in seven children diagnosed with sleep terrors or somnambulism [97]. Paroxetine at a dose of 40 mg in the morning was used successfully in a 46-year-old woman with a 30-year history of sleep terrors and somnambulism. REM suppressant properties of the antidepressants would appear to be a rational approach to the control of nightmares, though the evidence is not convincing [98]. Given these therapeutic uncertainties with use of the antidepressants for parasomnias and sleep related movement disorders, these drug classes are not first line treatments for these disorders and will not be discussed in depth here.

8. The alpha 2 delta subunit neuronal voltage-gated calcium channel blockers

The two drugs in this class are gabapentin and pregabalin and will be discussed separately. These drugs are not used for management of parasomnias, but have gained increasing favor for use in restless legs syndrome and periodic limb movement disorder. The current recommendations of the Scientific and Medical Advisory Board of the Restless Legs Syndrome Foundation were recently published in Mayo Clinic Proceedings. The alpha 2 delta subunit neuronal voltage-gated calcium channel blockers were recommended as first line therapy for chronic persistent restless legs syndrome (RLS) [99].

8.1 Gabapentin

Gabapentin was approved in December 1993 by the Food and Drug Administration (FDA) for the adjunctive therapy of partial seizures. After initial approval gabapentin sales increased significantly due to off-label uses for treatment of chronic pain syndromes [100]. In 2000 gabapentin was the top-selling anticonvulsant and ranked 17th in total expenditures among all drugs. In 2002 the FDA added the indication of postherpetic neuralgia, but by 2004 gabapentin sales had increased to 3 billion dollars per year [101]. In 2004 the US Department of Justice issued its largest fine to date ($430 million) to the Warner-Lambert group of pharmaceutical companies, manufacturer of gabapentin, for promoting gabapentin for uses not approved by the FDA [102]. In 2012 gabapentin enacarbil (a pro-drug with better absorption characteristics) received FDA approval for the treatment of restless legs syndrome and postherpetic neuralgia. By 2015 the use of gabapentin formulations had tripled from 2002 [103]. In 2017 gabapentin was the fifth most commonly prescribed medication in the United States [104].

Gabapentin has many desirable pharmacokinetic properties [105]. Mean maximum plasma concentrations were attained 2–3 hours after a 300–400 mg oral dose with a bioavailability of 60%, however, absorption kinetics are slowed and bioavailability decreased as the dose is increased. Gabapentin readily crosses the blood brain barrier due to its lipid solubility. It is not bound to plasma proteins. The elimination half-life is dependent on renal clearance alone in a linear fashion. The drug does not affect the metabolism of other drugs or induce hepatic enzymes. The elimination half-life of gabapentin after a single oral dose of 200–400 mg is about 5–7 hours with 80% of the dose recoverable unchanged in the urine. The most common adverse effects (significantly greater than placebo) are somnolence, dizziness, and ataxia. Happe et al. [106] reported efficacy of gabapentin given 2 hours before bedtime in restless legs syndrome in 2001. Subsequently, gabapentin enacarbil was found to be effective in a double-blind, placebo-controlled, multicenter study of 325 subjects [107]. This pro-drug (rapidly converted to gabapentin after absorption) sought to overcome the absorption deficiencies of gabapentin which was dependent upon active transport by a low-capacity nutrient transport system expressed in a narrow region of the upper small intestine. Gabapentin enacarbil is actively transported by a high-capacity nutrient transporter located throughout the large and small intestine [108]. There was significant improvement in RLS symptoms with both the 600 mg and 1200 mg doses of gabapentin enacarbil in the 12-week study compared to placebo. The most commonly reported adverse effects were dizziness and somnolence. Gabapentin enacarbil remains a preferable drug to generic gabapentin, however, cost concerns have made generic gabapentin more widely prescribed.

8.2 Pregabalin

Pregabalin and gabapentin share the same mechanism of action, inhibiting calcium influx into neuronal terminals and thus inhibiting the release of excitatory neurotransmitters. Orally dosed pregabalin is absorbed more rapidly than gabapentin with maximal plasma concentrations achieved in 1 hour [108]. The absorption is linear with plasma concentrations increasing proportionally to dose and the bioavailability of 90% or greater. Neither drug binds to plasma proteins or inhibits hepatic enzymes, and both drugs are eliminated by renal excretion alone with elimination half-lives of less than 6 hours. At higher dose therapy (1800–4800 mg) gabapentin bioavailability can fall to 25–50% [109]. Pregabalin bioavailability remained above 90% across its entire dose range.

A randomized, double-blind, 6-week study of pregabalin in 137 patients with restless legs syndrome showed an effective daily dose for 50% of patients at 37.3 mg and for 90% of patients at 123.9 mg per day [110]. A higher proportion of responders to the Clinical Global Impressions-Improvement Scale (CGI-I) was seen at the two highest doses of pregabalin 300 and 450 mg per day. Dizziness and somnolence were the most common adverse effects, though dry mouth complaints also exceeded placebo. A second double-blind, placebo-controlled study [111] was performed almost simultaneously with the Allen et al. [110] study. This second study randomized 58 patients in a 12-week flexible-dose trial. The mean effective dose at the end of treatment was 322.5 mg per day. There was a significant improvement in the International Restless Legs Scale (IRLS) and Clinical Global Impression (CGI). Polysomnography measured a reduction in mean periodic limb movement index, improvement in sleep architecture, and decrease in wakefulness after sleep onset. Adverse effects were reported to be mild and included unsteadiness, somnolence, and headache.

From the earliest studies of pregabalin there has been a concern about cognitive effects of this drug. Salinsky et al. [112] looked at this potential adverse effect in 32 healthy volunteers. The participants were randomized in a double-blind, parallel study receiving either pregabalin or placebo. Pregabalin was titrated over 8 weeks to 600 mg per day. At baseline and after 12 weeks of treatment all subjects underwent cognitive testing. A battery of 14 tests were used including finger tapping, grooved pegboard, digit symbol, Stroop color-word, selective reminding, name learning, story recall, Wonderlic personnel, visual reaction time, controlled oral word association, divided attention, letter-number sequencing, profile of mood states and Portland neurotoxicity scale. Thirty subjects completed the trial. There was significant ($p < 0.01$) worsening in the treatment group on the objective Stroop-color-word test and controlled oral word association test, as well as, the subjective Portland neurotoxicity scale. While the study demonstrated cognitive effects, both the speed of the titration and the final dose were greater than this author's current practice and the methodology of the treatment studies described here. This study, however, does demonstrate concerns over rapid dose increases and high dose therapy.

9. The dopamine receptor agonists

The dopamine agonists have been the first line treatment of periodic limb movement disorder and restless legs syndrome for many years. It is only recently that the alpha 2 delta subunit neuronal voltage-gated calcium channel blockers have advanced to preferred therapy [99]. It has, however, been long appreciated that the dopamine receptor agonists have adverse effects [113]. Impulse control disorders such as pathological gambling, hypersexuality, compulsive shopping, or an irresistible urge to wander have been identified in surveys [114]. The D3 dopamine receptor has been implicated in these behaviors [115], however, no dose response curve or dose related risk assessment has been established for these phenomena. A more pervasive and widespread adverse effect is the phenomena of augmentation. Augmentation manifests as earlier onset of RLS symptoms with decreased duration of benefit from medications and symptoms involving other parts of the body. Though the highest risk of augmentation occurs with short acting agents such as levodopa, current expert opinion is that augmentation will occur with all the currently available dopamine agonists over time [99].

9.1 Pramipexole

Pramipexole is a non-ergot dopamine agonist with higher affinity to D3 than D2 or D4 receptor subtypes. It has FDA indications for Parkinson's disease and restless leg syndrome [116]. It is rapidly absorbed and reaches peak plasma concentrations in 2 hours. If taken with a meal the absorption is delayed by about an hour. The bioavailability of pramipexole is greater than 90%. Renal excretion is the primary route of elimination with 90% of the dose recovered unchanged in the urine. The half-life of pramipexole is 8 hours in young adults and 12 hours in the elderly. The most common adverse effect (in excess of placebo) was somnolence. The recommended final treatment dose after up-titration was 0.5 mg given 2–3 hours before bedtime. Though higher doses are used in practice, the risk of increasing augmentation with high dose therapy leads to concern about high dosing [68].

9.2 Rotigotine

Rotigotine is dispensed as a transdermal delivery system [117]. It is a non-ergoline dopamine agonist for the D3, D2, and D1 dopamine receptors approved by the FDA for use in RLS as well as Parkinson's disease. When a patch is applied there is a 3-hour delay before the drug is detected in plasma and the time to maximal plasm levels is 15–18 hours. Approximately 45% of the dose is released from the patch in 24 hours. After removal of the patch the elimination half-life is 5–7 hours. Most rotigotine is eliminated in the urine as inactive conjugates. The highest recommended dose (for RLS) of rotigotine is 3 mg per 24 hours. The most common adverse effect was a skin reaction at the site of the patch, though nausea also exceeded placebo. The constant delivery system suppresses RLS augmentation temporarily though other medications may ultimately be needed for breakthrough symptoms [68].

9.3 Ropinirole

Ropinirole is a selective non-ergoline dopamine D3 much greater than D2 receptor agonist [118]. It is rapidly absorbed but its bioavailability is only 50%. The maximal plasma concentrations are achieved in 0.5 to 4 hours (mean 1.5 hours). The drug is metabolized in the liver to inactive metabolites by the P450 iso-enzyme CYP1A2. The elimination half-life is 3 hours, though this can be variable and elderly patients have 15% slower clearance. The drug is FDA approved for use in restless legs syndrome, as well as, Parkinson's disease. The short half-life and duration of action of this drug can lead to tachyphylaxis and doses higher than recommended producing a high rate of augmentation in the author's experience.

10. Prazosin

The American Academy of Sleep Medicine published a position paper on the treatment of nightmare disorder in 2018 [119]. The position paper divided nightmares into those associated with post-traumatic stress disorder (PTSD) and those not associated with PTSD. Nightmares associated with PTSD are more difficult to suppress and thus a wide variety of behavioral and drug combinations have been used, beyond the capability of this chapter. The drugs that may be used in nightmare disorder in the absence of PTSD are benzodiazepines, not including clonazepam, and prazosin.

Prazosin is a quinazoline derivative and peripheral vasodilator [120]. Its vasodilator properties are due to postsynaptic alpha adrenergic receptor blockade. Prazosin is extensively metabolized in the liver producing high first pass elimination and resultant low oral bioavailability after oral dosing. With an oral dose of 1 mg in normal subjects the bioavailability of prazosin ranged from 43.5 to 69.3% [121]. The mean elimination half-life is about 2.5 hours. Prazosin shows initial dose postural hypotension which disappears with continued administration.

On acute administration of prazosin, only very low levels crossed the blood–brain barrier [122]. On chronic administration of high dose prazosin, however, prazosin apparently crossed the blood–brain barrier in adequate concentrations to affect the central alpha adrenergic receptor density in the cerebral cortex [123]. This effect would not have occurred without significant penetration of prazosin into the brain. There were a number of studies showing efficacy of prazosin in veterans with PTSD induced nightmares [119]. In contrast, however, there was a recent large randomized, placebo-controlled study with negative results [124], leading to uncertainty about this treatment.

11. The opioids

Various opioids have been used for intractable restless legs syndrome. These include propoxyphene [125]. tramadol [126], oxycodone [127], hydrocodone [128], and methadone [129]. Most of these have been used as adjunctive therapy, but methadone has been used in monotherapy. The mechanism of action of the opioids in RLS is unclear, however, it appears to work through a central dopaminergic neurotransmission as dopamine receptor antagonists will block the therapeutic effect. The current opioid crisis has lent a stigma to chronic use of methadone that has discouraged its use by many patients suffering with intractable restless legs syndrome. This is unfortunate as opioid therapy with management directed towards restless legs syndrome rather than chronic pain syndromes can be quite helpful [130]. The concern with long-term opioid therapy is the occult development or exacerbation of a sleep related breathing disorder. For this reason, all patients on chronic opioids should be clinically monitored for evidence of sleep apnea [131].

11.1 Methadone

Methadone is a synthetic opioid that is nearly equipotent with morphine, but with dramatically different pharmacokinetic characteristics [132]. Methadone is a racemic mixture of R and S-methadone with the R isomer being 8–50 times more potent. Methadone may prevent or attenuate opioid tolerance via its weak antagonist properties on the N-methyl-D-aspartate (NMDA) receptor. Methadone is rapidly absorbed with maximal plasma concentrations 2.5 to 4 hours after oral administration. The bioavailability of methadone is 70–80%, though this can vary depending on the degree of first pass metabolism. Methadone is hepatically metabolized to inactive metabolites by the cytochrome P450 enzymes, CYP3A4 and CYP2B6. The elimination half-life of methadone ranges from 5 to 130 hours with a mean of 20–35 hours. The elimination half-life of the R isomer is approximately 25% longer than the S isomer. Methadone shows apparent autoinduction of its own metabolism. The half-life during chronic therapy is only 40% of the half-life with acute administration. A number of medications can either decrease or increase methadone levels via induction or inhibition of CYP3A4. Quantitative plasma levels may be necessary. Of note, there have been unintentional deaths with methadone. Many of these deaths occurred on the fifth day of regular dosing [133]. Prescribers need to be aware of methadone's peculiar pharmacokinetics.

In practice doses of methadone from 5–40 mg daily have been used. Given the pharmacokinetics starting therapy at a small dose of 2.5–5 mg is appropriate with up-titration of the dose as needed for symptoms. Methadone in patients with intractable RLS can produce remarkable improvement [68, 129].

11.2 Oxycodone-naloxone

Constipation and bowel dysfunction is the prime adverse effect of long-term opiate therapy. The combination of an opioid with a competitive mu receptor antagonist in a sustained release formulation is a unique answer to opioid adverse effects. The combination is also a tool against abuse of oxycodone since dissolution and injection results in naloxone having a much greater effect blocking mu receptors. A double-blind, randomized, placebo-controlled trial with this formulation was performed with 276 RLS patients [134]. The study started participants on a dose of oxycodone 5.0 mg and naloxone 2.5 mg twice a day increasing per each study site's investigator to a maximal dose of oxycodone 40 mg and naloxone 20 mg. Adverse effects more than twice as frequent as placebo included fatigue, constipation, somnolence, dry mouth and pruritis. There was clear efficacy of the combination over placebo.

12. Conclusions

This chapter did not attempt to be all inclusive, as a full description of the pharmacological interventions into sleep related movement disorders and parasomnias would fill the entire book. The chapter does attempt to provide pharmacological basis for treatment of the most challenging areas for pharmaceutical intervention, notably the REM sleep parasomnias and restless legs syndrome.

A challenge of REM sleep parasomnia management is the continuing use of clonazepam as first line therapy. This potent drug is effective, but due to its extremely long half-life, is prone to adverse effects in many patients. Unfortunately, the even more potent drug, triazolam, is too short acting and the two drugs (alprazolam and lorazepam) with duration of actions that are reasonable for the goal of suppressing dream enactment are less potent than either triazolam or clonazepam, thus appearing to need higher doses. Unexpectedly, the observational experience of the University of Texas Southwestern Medical Center at Dallas Clinical Center for Sleep and Breathing Disorders has been that the efficacy of alprazolam is half the expected dose that was used in trials in Minneapolis. Retrospective review is in progress.

The other pharmacological challenge is the management of severe persistent and intractable restless leg syndrome. In recent decades the algorithms for management have become clearer pointing to the early use of gabapentin and pregabalin and the use of opioids in intractable patients, however, there is a lag of that knowledge reaching the medical community that is faced with these patients and their demands for treatment. This is another area where the growth of medical knowledge is exceeding our educational capabilities.

Author details

Gregory S. Carter
The University of Texas Southwestern Medical Center at Dallas, Dallas, Texas, United States of America

*Address all correspondence to: gregory.carter@utsouthwestern.edu

References

[1] Roger H. Les Troubles du Sommeil. Paris: Masson; 1932 p. 275-283

[2] American Academy of Sleep Medicine. Parasomnias. In: AASM, ed. International Classification of Sleep Disorders, 3rd Edition. Darien: American Academy of Sleep Medicine; 2014. p. 225-280

[3] American Academy of Sleep Medicine. Sleep-related movement disorders. In: AASM, ed. International Classification of Sleep Disorders, 3rd Ed. Darien: American Academy of Sleep Medicine; 2014. p. 281-337

[4] Ohayon MM. Epidemiology of parasomnias. In: Thorpy MJ and Plazzi G, editors. Parasomnias and Other Sleep-Related Movement Disorders. New York: Cambridge University Press; 2010. p. 301-311

[5] Gulyani S, Salas RE, and Gamaldo CE. Sleep medicine pharmacotherapeutics overview: Today, tomorrow, and the future (Part 2: hypersomnia, parasomnia, and movement disorders). Chest. 2013. 143(1): 242-251

[6] Klackenberg G. Somnambulism in childhood-prevalence, course and behavioral correlations: a prospective longitudinal study (3-16 years). Acta Paediatr Scand. 1982; 71:495-499

[7] Simonds J and Parraga H. Prevalence of sleep disorders and sleep behaviors in children and adolescents. J Am Acad Child Adolesc Psychiatry. 1982; 21:383-388

[8] Hublin C, Kaprio J, Partinen M, Heikkila K, Koskenvuo M. Parasomnias:co-occurrence and genetics. Psychiatr Genet. 2001; 11:65-70

[9] Lateef O, Wyatt J, and Cartwright R. A case of violent non-REM parasomnias that resolved with treatment of obstructive sleep apnea. Chest. 2005; 128(4 Meeting abstracts):461S

[10] Drakatos P, Marples L, Muza R, Higgins S, Gildeh N, Macavei R, Dongol EM, Nesbitt A, Rosenweig I, Lyons E, d'Ancona G, Steier J, Williams AJ and Kent BD. NREM parasomnis: a treatment approach based upon a retrospective case series of 512 patients. Sleep Med. 2018; 53(1):181-188

[11] Attarian H and Zhu L. Treatment options for disorders of arousal: a case series. Int J Neurosci. 2013;123(9):623-625

[12] Hauri PJ, Silber M, and Boeve BF. The treatment of parasomnias with hypnosis: a 5-year follow-up study. J Clin Sleep Med. 2007; 3(4):369-373.

[13] Proserpio P, Teraghi M, Manni R, and Nobili L. Drugs used in parasomnia. Sleep Medicine Clinics. 2020; 15(2):289-300

[14] Schenck CH, Milner TD, Hurwitz et.al. A polysomnographic and clinical report on sleep-related injury in 100 adult patients. Am J Psychiatry. 1989;146(9):1166-1173

[15] Schenk CH and Mahowald MW. Long-term, nightly benzodiazepine treatment of injurious parasomnias and other disorders of disrupted nocturnal sleep in 170 adults. Am J Med. 1996;100(3):333-337

[16] Goldbloom D and Chouinard G. Clonazepam in the treatment of neuroleptic-induced somnambulism. Am J Psychiatry. 1984;141(11):1486

[17] Nutt DH, Wilson SJ, Lillywhite AR, Potokar JP, and Bell CJ. Adult night terrors and paroxetine. Lancet. 1997;350(9072):185

[18] Cooper AJ. Treatment of coexistent night-terrors and somnambulism in adults with imipramine and diazepam. J Clin Psychiatry. 1987; 48(5):209-210

[19] Balon R. Sleep terror disorder and insomnia treated with trazodone: a case report. Ann Clin Psychiatry. 1994;6(3):161-163

[20] Jan JE, Freeman RD, Wasdell MB, and Bomben MM. A child with severe night terrors and sleep-walking responds to melatonin therapy. Dev Med Child Neurol. 2004;46(11):789

[21] Ozcan O and Donmez YE. Melatonin treatment for childhood sleep terror. J Child Adolesc Psychopharmacol. 2014;24(9):528-529

[22] van Zyl LT, Chung S., Shahid A, and Shapiro CM. L-Tryptophan as treatment for pediatric non-rapid eye movement parasomnia. J Child Adolesc Psychopharmacol. 2018; 28(6):395-401

[23] Bruni O, Ferri R, Miano S, et.al. L-5-hydroxytryptophan treatment of sleep terrors in children. Eur J Pediatr. 2004; 163(7):402-407

[24] Sasayma D, Washizuka S, and Honda H. Effective treatment of night terrors and sleep walking with ramelteon. J Child Adolesc Psychopharmacol. 2016;26(10):948

[25] Guilleminault C and Silvestri JM. Disorders of arousal and epilepsy during sleep. In: Sterman M, Shouse M, Passouant P, editors. Sleep and Epilepsy. New York: Academic Press; 1983. p. 513-531

[26] Tung L and Carter G. Differentiating confusional parasomnias from nocturnal frontal lobe epilepsy. Sleep 2019; 42(Abstract Suppl): A425-A426

[27] Montini A, Loddo G, Balelli L, Cilea R, and Provini F. Sleep-related hypermotor epilepsy vs disorders of arousal in adults. A step-wise approach to diagnosis. Chest. 2021; 160(1):319-329

[28] Fleetham JA, Jonathan AE, and Fleming MB. Parasomnias. Canadian Medical Association Journal. 2014;186(8): E273-E280

[29] Haba-Rubio J, Frauscher B, Marques-Vidal P, Toriel J, Tobback N, Andries D, Preisig M, Vollenweider P, Postuma R, and Heinzer R. Prevalence and determinants of REM sleep behavior disorder in the general population. Sleep. 2018; 41(2):1-8

[30] McKenna and Peever J. REM sleep behavior disorder: The link between synucleinopathies and REM sleep circuits. In: Rapid-Eye-Movement Sleep Behavior Disorder, Schenck CH, Högl B, and Videnovic A, editors. Cham: Springer Nature Switzerland AG; 2019. p. 625-637

[31] Iranzo A and Santamaria J. Severe obstructive sleep apnea/hypopnea mimicking REM sleep behavior disorder. Sleep. 2005; 28:203-206

[32] Olson E, Boeve B, and Silber M. Rapid eye movement sleep behavior disorder: demographic, clinical, and laboratory findings in 93 cases. Brain. 2000; 123:331-339

[33] Levin R and Fireman G. Nightmare prevalence, nightmare distress, and self-reported psychological disturbance. Sleep. 2002; 25:205-212

[34] Germain A and Nielsen T. Sleep pathophysiology in posttraumatic stress disorder and idiopathic nightmare suffers. Biol. Psychiatry. 2003; 54:1092-1098

[35] Pagel J and Helfter P. Drug induced nightmares-an etiology-based review. Hum Psychopharmacol. 2003; 18:59-67

[36] Brooks LJ and Topol HI. Enuresis in children with sleep apnea. J Pediatr. 2003; 142:515-518

[37] Held-Egli K, Ruegger C, Das-Kundu S, Schmitt B, Bucher HU. Benign neonatal sleep myoclonus in new born infants of opioid dependent mothers. Acta Paediatr. 2009; 98:69-73

[38] Lavigne G, Guitard F, Rompre P, Montplaisir J. Variability in sleep bruxism activity over time. J Sleep Res. 2001; 10:237-244

[39] Ohayon M, Li K, and Guilleminault C, Risk factors for sleep bruxism in the general population. Chest. 2001; 119:53-61

[40] Ondo WG, Simmons JH, Shahid MH, Hashem V, Hunter C, and Jankovic J. Onabotulinum toxin-A injections for sleep bruxism: A double-blind, placebo-controlled study. Neurology. 2018; 90(7): e559-e564

[41] Shim YJ, Lee HJ, Park KJ, Kim HT, Hong IH, and Kim ST. Botulinum toxin therapy for managing sleep bruxism: A randomized and placebo-controlled trial. Toxins. 2020;12(3):168-177

[42] Butler J, Mulkerrin E, and O'Keefe S. Nocturnal leg cramps in older people. Postgrad Med J 2002; 78:596-598

[43] Weiner I and Weiner H. Nocturnal leg muscle cramps. JAMA. 1980; 244:2332-2333

[44] Iber C, Ancoli-Israel S, Chesson AL Jr., and Quan SF for the American Academy of Sleep Medicine. The AASM Manual for the Scoring of Sleep and Associated Events: Rules, Terminology and Technical Specifications, First Edition: Westchester, Illinois: American Academy of Sleep Medicine, 2007

[45] Baenninger A. Good Chemistry: The Life and Legacy of Valium Inventor Leo Sternbach. New York: McGraw-Hill; 2003. 256 p

[46] Ciraulo DA and Oldham M. Sedative hypnotics. In: The Effects of Drug Abuse on the Human Nervous System. Madras B and Kuhar M, editors. 2014. Boston: Elsevier BV; 2011. p. 499-532

[47] Jick H, Miettinen OS, Shapiro S, Lewis GP. Comprehensive drug surveillance. JAMA. 1970; 213:1455-1460

[48] Gable RS. Toward a comparative overview of dependance potential and acute toxicity of psychoactive substances used nonmedically. Am J Drug Alcohol Abuse. 1993; 19:263-281

[49] Drug Enforcement Administration. Benzodiazepines (Street Names: Benzos, Downers, Nerve Pills, Tranks). December 2019. Drug and Chemical Evaluation Section https://www.deadiversion.usdoj.gov/drug_chem_info/benzo.pdf [Accessed 2021-08-16]

[50] National Institute on Drug Abuse. Trends and Statistics. https://www.drugabuse.gov/drug-topics/trends-statistics/overdose-death-rates [Accessed 2021-08-16]

[51] DeVane CL. Clinical pharmacokinetics and pharmacodynamics of anxiolytics and sedative/hypnotics. In: Jann M, Penzak S, and Cohen L, editors. Applied Clinical Pharmacokinetics and Pharmacodynamics of Psychopharmacological Agents. Adis, Cham: Springer. 2016. p. 1-39. https:// doi.org/10.1007/978-3-319-27883-4_10

[52] Bergman R, Kongsbak K, Sorensen PL, Sander T, and Balle T. A unified model of the GABA-A receptor comprising agonist and benzodiazepine binding sites. PLos One. 2013;8(1): e52323. doi: 10.1371/journal.pone.0052323

[53] Collinson N, Kuenzi EM, Jarolimek W, Maubach KA, Cothliff R, Sur C, Smith A, Otu FM, Howell O, Atack JR, McKernan RM, Seabrook GR, Dawson GR, Whiting PJ, and Rosahl TW. Enhanced learning and memory and altered GABAergic synaptic transmission in mice lacking the alpha 5 subunit of the $GABA_A$ receptor. J Neurosci. 2002; 22(13):5572-5580

[54] Kralic JE, Korpi ER, O'Buckley TK, Homanics GE, and Morrow AL. Molecular and pharmacological characterization of GABA(A) receptor alpha1 subunit knockout mice. J Pharmacol Exp Ther. 2002; 302(3):1037-1045

[55] Greenblatt DJ and Wright CW. Clinical pharmacokinetics of alprazolam. Therapeutic implications. Clin Pharmacokinet, 1993;24(6): 453-471

[56] Lasher TA, Fleishaker JC, Steenwyk RC, and Antal EJ. Pharmacokinetic pharmacodynamic evaluation of the combined administration of alprazolam and fluoxetine. Psychopharmacol. 1991; 104:323-327

[57] Greenblatt DJ, Divoli M, Abernathy DR, Moschitto LJ, Smith RB, et.al. Alprazolam kinetics in the elderly. Relation to antipyrine disposition. Arch Gen Psychiatry. 1983; 40:287-290

[58] Arendt RM, Greenblatt DJ, Liebisch DC, Luu MD, and Paul SM. Determinants of benzodiazepine brain uptake: lipophilicity versus binding affinity. Psychopharmacol. 1987; 93:7276

[59] Dehlin O, Kullingsjö H, Lidén A, Agrell B, Moser G, Olsen I. Pharmacokinetics of alprazolam in geriatric patients with neurotic depression. Basic Clin Pharmacol Toxicol. 1991; 68:121-124

[60] Ktoboth PD, McAuley JW, and Smith RB. Alprazolam in the elderly: pharmacokinetics and pharmacodynamics during multiple dosing. Psychopharmacol. 1990; 100:477-484

[61] Wright CE and Chambers JH. Influence of alprazolam input rate and steady-state pharmacokinetics on psychomotor performance in healthy subjects. Pharm Res. 1991; 8:250

[62] Garzone PD and Kroboth PD. Pharmacokinetics of the newer benzodiazepines. Clin Pharmacokinet. 1989; 16:337-364

[63] Dobbs FR, Banks W, Fleishaker JC, Valentine AD, Kinsey BM, Franceschini MP, Digenis GA, and Tewson TJ. Studies with [11C] alprazolam: an agonist for the benzodiazepine receptor. Nucl Med Biol 1995; 22(4): 459-466

[64] Miller LG, Greenblatt DJ, Barnhill JG, Deutsch SL, Shader RI, and Paul SM. Benzodiazepine receptor binding of triazolobenzodiazepines in vivo: increased receptor number with low-dose alprazolam. J Neurochem. 1987; 49:1595-1601

[65] Aurora RN, Zak RS, Maganti RK, Auerbach SH, Casey KR, Chowdhuri S, Karippot A, Ramar K, Kristo DA, and Morgenthaler TI. Best Practice Guide for the Treatment of REM Sleep Behavior Disorder (RBD). J Clin Sleep Med. 2010; 6(1): 85-95

[66] Schenck CH, Boyd JL, and Mahowald MW. A parasomnia overlap disorder involving sleepwalking, sleep terrors, and REM sleep behavior disorder in 33 polysomnographically confirmed cases. Sleep 1997; 20:972-981

[67] Schenck CH and Mahowald MW. Long-term, nightly benzodiazepine treatment of injurious parasomnias and other disorders of disrupted nocturnal

sleep in 170 adults. Am J Med. 1996; 100:333-337

[68] Carter GS. Unpublished data. UT Southwestern. 2021. Dallas Texas

[69] Patel A and Carter, G. Electrocution as a rare cause of REM sleep behavior disorder. Sleep. 2019; 42(Abstract Suppl): A417

[70] Altamura AC, M. D., Paletta S, Maffini M, Mauri MC, and Bareggi S. Understanding the pharmacokinetics of anxiolytic drugs. Expert Opin Drug Metab Toxicol. 2013; 9(4):423-440.

[71] Sher PK and Machen VL. Benzodiazepine receptor affinity alterations at physiologic temperature after chronic clonazepam exposure. Brain Dev 1987; 9:33-36

[72] Galpern WR, Lumpkin M, Greenblatt DJ, Shader RI, and Miller LG. Chronic benzodiazepine administration. VII. Behavioral tolerance and withdrawal and receptor alterations associated with clonazepam administration. Psychopharmacol. 1991; 104:225-230

[73] Ellinwood EH, Nikaido AM, Gupta SK, Heatherly DG, and Hege S. Comparison of the relationship between structure and CNS effects for lorazepam, clonazepam and alprazolam. J Psychopharm. 1993; 7(1):24-32

[74] Ciraulo DA and Oldham M (2014). Sedative hypnotics. In: The Effects of Drug Abuse on the Human Nervous System. Madras B and Kuhar M, editors, New York: Elsevier; 2014. p. 499-532.

[75] Boeve BF, Silber MH, and Ferman TJ. Melatonin for treatment of REM sleep behavior disorder in neurologic disorders: results in 14 patients. Sleep Med. 2003; 4:281-284

[76] Antón-Tay F, Días JL, and Fernández-Guardiola A. On the effect of melatonin upon the human brain. Its possible therapeutic implications. Life Sci-Part I-Physiol Pharmacol 1971; 10:841-850

[77] Lieberman HR, Waldhauser F, Garfield G, Lynch HJ, and Wurtman RJ. Effects of melatonin on human mood and performance. Brain Res. 1984; 323:201-207

[78] Buscemi N, Vandermeer B, Hooton N, Pandya R, Tjosvold L, Hartling L, Baker G, Klassen TP, and Vohra S. The efficacy and safety of exogenous melatonin for primary sleep disorders. A meta-analysis. J Gen Intern Med. 2005; 20:1151-1158

[79] Moroni I, Garcia-Bennett A, Chapman J, Grunstein RR, Gordon CJ, and Comas M. Pharmacokinetics of exogenous melatonin in relation to formulation, and effects on sleep: A systematic review. Sleep Med Rev. 2021; 57:101431 https://doi.org/10.1016/j.smrv.2021.101431

[80] Facciolá G, Hidestrand M, von Bahr C, and Tybring G. Cytochrome P-450 isoforms involved in melatonin metabolism in human liver microsomes. Eur J Clin Pharmacol. 2001; 56(12):881-888

[81] Ma X, Idle JR, Krausz KW, and Gonzalez FJ. Metabolism of melatonin by human cytochromes P450. Drug Metabol Dispos. 2005; 33(4):489-494

[82] Fourtillan JB, Brisson AM, Gobin P, Ingrand I, Decourt JP and Girault J. Bioavailability of melatonin in humans after day-time administration of D(7) melatonin. Biopharm Drug Dispos. 2000; 21(1):15-22

[83] Zhdanova IV, Wurtman RJ, Balcioglu A, Kartashov AI, and Lynch HJ. Endogenous melatonin levels and the fate of exogenous melatonin: age effects. J Gerontol Series A, Biol Sci Med Sci. 1998; 53(4):8293-8298

[84] Proserpio P, Terzaghi M, Manni R, and Nobili L. Drugs used in parasomnia. Sleep Med Clin. 2020;15(2):289-300

[85] Auger RR, Burgess HJ, Emens JS, Deriy LV, Thomas SM, Sharkey KM. Clinical practice guideline for the treatment of intrinsic circadian rhythm sleep-wake disorders: advanced sleep-wake phase disorder (ASWPD), delayed sleep-wake phase disorder (DSWPD), non-24-hour sleep-wake rhythm disorder (N24SWD), and irregular sleep-wake rhythm disorder (ISWRD). An update for 2015. J Clin Sleep Med. 2015; 11(10):1199-1236

[86] Werneke U, Turner T, and Priebe S. Complementary medicines in psychiatry: review of effectiveness and safety. Br J Psychiatry; 2006; 188:109-121

[87] Rubio-Sastre P, Scheer FA, Gómez-Abellán P, Madrid JA, Garaulet M. Acute melatonin administration in humans impairs glucose tolerance in both the morning and evening. Sleep; 2014; 37:1715-1719

[88] Luboshitzky R, Shen-Orr Z, Nave R, Lavi S, and Lavie P. Melatonin administration alters semen quality in healthy men. J Androl; 2002; 23:572-578

[89] Valcavi R, Zini M, Maestroni GJ, Conti A, and Portioli I. Melatonin stimulates growth hormone secretion through pathways other than the growth hormone-releasing hormone. Clin Endocrinol; 1993; 39:193-199.

[90] Kierlin L and Littner MR. Parasomnias and antidepressant therapy: a review of the literature. Frontiers in Psychiatry. 2011; 2:71,1-71,8

[91] Winkelman J and James L. Serotonergic antidepressants are associated with REM sleep without atonia. Sleep. 2004; 27:317-321

[92] Teman PT, Tippmann-Peikert M, Silber M, Slocumb NL, and Auger RR. Idiopathic rapid-eye-movement sleep disorder: associations with antidepressants, psychiatric diagnoses, and other factors, in relation to the age of onset. Sleep Med. 2009; 10:60-65

[93] Yeh Y, Chen C, Feng H, Wang SC, Kuo SC, and Chen CK. New onset somnambulism associated with different dosage of mirtazapine: a case report. Clin Neuropharmacol. 2009; 32:232-233

[94] Hoque R and Chesson AL. Pharmacologically induced/exacerbated restless legs syndrome, periodic limb movements of sleep, and REM behavior disorder/REM sleep without atonia: literature review, qualitative scoring, and comparative analysis. J Clin Sleep Med. 2010; 6:79-83

[95] Lam SP, Fong SY, Ho CK, Yu MW, and Wing YK. Parasomnia among psychiatric outpatients: clinical, epidemiologic, cross-sectional study. J Clin Psychiatry 2008; 69:1374-1382

[96] Pesikoff RB and Davis PC. Treatment of pavor nocturnus and somnambulism in children. Am J Psychiatry. 1971; 136: 1087-1088

[97] Lillywhite AR, Wilson SJ, and Nutt DJ. Successful treatment of night terrors and somnambulism with paroxetine. Br J Psychiatry. 1994; 164:551-554

[98] van Liempt S, Vermetten E, Geuze E, and Westenberg H. Pharmacotherapeutic treatment of nightmares and insomnia in posttraumatic stress disorder: an overview of the literature. Ann NY Acad Sci. 2006; 1071: 502-507

[99] Silber MH, Buchfuhrer MJ, Earley CJ, Koo BB, Manconi M, and Winkelman JW. The management of restless legs syndrome: an updated

algorithm. Mayo Clin Proc. 2021; 96(7):1921-1937

[100] Wallach JD and Ross JS. Gabapentin approvals, off-label use, and lessons for postmarketing evaluation efforts. JAMA. 2018; 319(8):776-778

[101] Landefeld CS and Steinman MA. The Neurontin legacy-marketing through misinformation and manipulation. N Engl J Med. 2009; 360(2):103-106

[102] Department of Justice. Warner-Lambert to pay $430 million to resolve criminal and civil health care liability related to off-label promotion. 2004 [press release]. https://www.justice.gov/archive/opa/pr/2004/May/04_civ_322.htm [Accessed 2021-08-15]

[103] Johansen ME. Gabapentinoid use in the United States 2002 through 2015. JAMA Intern Med.2018; doi:10.1001/jamainternmed.2017.7856

[104] GoodRx. The GoodRx top 10: July 2017. https://www.beckershospitalreview.com/supply-chain/10-most-popular-prescription-drugs-for-2017.html [Accessed 2021-08-16]

[105] Goa KL and Sorkin EM. Gabapentin. A review of its pharmacological properties and clinical potential in epilepsy. Drugs. 1993; 46(3):409-427

[106] Happe S, Klösch G, Saletu B, and Zeitlhofer J. Treatment of idiopathic restless legs syndrome (RLS) with gabapentin. Neurology. 2001; 57:1717-1719

[107] Lee DO, Ziman RB, Perkins T, Poceta JS, Walters AS, Barrett RW and the XP053 Study Group. A randomized, double-blind, placebo-controlled study to assess the efficacy and tolerability of gabapentin enacarbil in subjects with restless legs syndrome. J Clin Sleep Med. 2011; 7(3):282-292

[108] Cundy KC, Branch R, Chernov-Rogan T, Dias T, Estrada T, Hold K, Koller K, Liu X, Mann A, Panuwat M, Raillard SP, Upadhyay S, Wu QQ, Xiang Jia-Ning, Yan Hui, Zerangue N, Zhou CX, Barrett RW, and Gallop MA. XP13512, a novel gabapentin prodrug: I. Design, synthesis, enzymatic conversion to gabapentin, and transport by intestinal solute transporters. J Pharmacol Exp Ther. 2004; 311:315-323

[109] Wilson EA, Sills GJ, Forrest G, Brodie MJ. High dose gabapentin in refractory partial epilepsy: clinical observations in 50 patients. Epilepsy Res. 1998; 29(2): 161-166

[110] Allen R, Chen C, Soaita A, Wohlberg C, Knapp L, Peterson BT, García-Borreguero D, and Miceli J. A randomized, double-blind, 6-week, dose-ranging study of pregabalin in patients with restless legs syndrome. Sleep Med. 2010; 11:512-519

[111] García-Borreguero D, Larrosa O, Williams A-M, Albares J, Pascual M, Palacios JC, and Fernandez C. Treatment of restless legs syndrome with pregabalin. A double-blind, placebo-controlled study. Neurology. 2010; 74:1897-1904

[112] Salinsky M, Storzbach D, and Munoz S. Cognitive effects of pregabalin in healthy volunteers. A double-blind, placebo-controlled trial. Neurology. 2010; 74:755-761

[113] Silber MH and Allen RP. Dopaminergic therapy of restless leg syndrome. In: Hening WA, Chokroverty S, Allen RP, and Earley CJ. Editors. Restless Legs Syndrome. Philadelphia: Saunders Elsevier; 2009. p. 238-254

[114] Moore TJ, Glenmullen J, and Mattison DR. Reports of pathological

gambling, hypersexuality, and compulsive shopping associated with dopamine receptor agonist drugs. JAMA Intern Med. 2014; 174(12):1930-1933

[115] Kelley BJ, Duker AP, and Chiu P. Dopamine agonists and pathological behaviors. Parkinson's Disease. 2012; doi:10.1155/2012/603631

[116] Boehringer Ingelheim. Mirapex (pramipexole dihydrochloride) Prescribing information. 2007. http://us.boehringer-ingelheim.com [Accessed 2021-08-13]

[117] Schwartz Pharma, LLC. Neupro (Rotigotine transdermal system) 2012 https://www.accessdata.fda.gov/drugsatfda_docs/label/2012/021829s001lbl.pdf [Accessed 2021-08-13]

[118] Kaye CM and Nicholls B. Clinical pharmacokinetics of ropinirole. Clin Pharmacokinet. 2000; 39(4):243-254

[119] Morgenthaler TI, Auerbach S, Casey KR, Kristo D, Maganti R, Ramar K, Zak R, and Kartje R. Position paper for the treatment of nightmare disorder in adults: an American Academy of Sleep Medicine Position Paper. J Clin Sleep Med. 2018;14(6):1041-1055

[120] Jaillon P. Clinical pharmacokinetics of prazosin. Clin Pharmacokinet. 1980; 5:365-376

[121] Bateman DN, Hobbs DC, Twomey TM, Stevens EA and Rawlins MD. Prazosin pharmacokinetics and concentration effect. Eur J Clin Pharmacol. 1979; 16:177-181

[122] Taylor JA, Twomey TM and Schach von Wittenau M. The metabolic fate of prazosin. Xenobiotica.1977; 7(6):357-364

[123] Takita M, Taniguchi T, Zhu J, and Muramatsu I. Chronic treatment with prazosin causes a subtype-specific increase in the alpha-1-adenoceptor density of the stressed rat cerebral cortex. J Pharm Pharmacol. 1997; 49:802-805

[124] Raskind MA, Peskind ER, Chow B, Harris C, Davis-Karim A, Holmes HA, Hart KL, McFall M, Mellman, TA, Reist C, Romesser J, Rosenheck R, Shih M-C, Stein MB, Swift R, Gleason T, Lu Y, and Huang GD. Trial of prazosin for post-traumatic stress disorder in military veterans. N Eng J Med. 2018; 378(6):507-517

[125] Kaplan PW, Allen RP, Buchholz DW, and Walters JK. A double-blind, placebo-controlled study of the treatment of periodic limb movements in sleep using carbidopa/levodopa and propoxyphene. Sleep. 1993; 16:717-723

[126] Lauerma H and Markkula J. Treatment of restless legs syndrome with tramadol: An open study. J Clin Psychiatry. 1999; 60:241-244

[127] Walters AS, Wagner ML, Hening WA, Grasing K, Mills R, Chokoverty S and Kavey N. Successful treatment of the idiopathic restless legs syndrome in a randomized double-blind trial of oxycodone versus placebo. Sleep. 1993; 16:327-332

[128] Kavey N, Walters AS, Hening W, and Gidro-Frank S. Opioid treatment of periodic movements in sleep in patients without restless legs. Neuropeptides. 1988; 11:181-184

[129] Ondo WC. Methadone for refractory restless legs syndrome. Mov Disord. 2005; 20:345-348

[130] Becker PM. Opioid agents in the treatment of restless legs syndrome. In: Hening WA, Chokroverty S, Allen RP, and Earley CJ. Editors. Restless Legs Syndrome. Philadelphia: Saunders Elsevier; 2009. p. 255-261

[131] Walters AS, Winkelman J, Trenkwalder C, Fry JM, Kataria V, Wagner M, Sharma R, Hening W, and Li L. Long-term follow-up on restless legs syndrome patients treated with opioids. Mov Disord. 2001; 16:1105-1109

[132] Lugo RA, Satterfield KL, and Kern SE. Pharmacokinetics of methadone. Journal of Pain & Palliative Care Pharmacotherapy. 2005;19(4):13-24

[133] Caravati EM, Grey T, Nangle B, Rolfs RT, and Peterson-Porucznik. Increase in poisoning deaths caused by illicit drugs-Utah, 1991-2003. MMWR Morb Mortal Wkly Rep. 2005; 54(2):33-36

[134] Trenkwalder C, Benes H, Grote L, Garcia-Borreguero D, Hogl B, Bosse, B, Oksche A, Reimer K, Winkelmann J, Allen RP, and Kohnen R. Prolonged release oxycodone-naloxone for treatment of severe restless legs syndrome after failure of previous treatment: a double-blind, randomized, placebo-controlled trial with an open-label extension. Lancet Neurol. 2013; 12:1141-1150

Section 3

Supplemental Interventional Modalities in Sleep Therapy

Chapter 5

Impact of Insomnia in the Elderly: The Correlation between Snoring and Apnea/Hypopnea Index

Bing Tang

Abstract

The purpose of this study was to examine the relationship between snoring and obstructive sleep apnea/hypopnea index in community dwelling older men and women. In this retrospective case-series study, the author was using a sequential collection of clinical datum design. There were 124 community-dwelling elders (mean age=71.85 years, Standard Deviation=4.85 years) with complaints of sleep disturbance. Including 46 females (F: M= 1:1.71), all the total subjects with sleep disturbance, after meeting the following criteria of exclusion: age below 65 years, heart failure, and chronic obstructive lung disease, were admitted to the sleep medicine laboratory where sleep questionnaire was used. They underwent in laboratory over-night polysomnography (PSG). The period of this study was 13 months; the total number of subjects whom took PSG in this Sleep Center Laboratory was 1,087 individuals during this period. The proposed neural model used is a generalized regression neural network (GRNN). This neural model has some advantages such as cost and time efficiencies in relation to experimental measurements. The training speed of the proposed technique is faster and the network architecture is simpler. In all likelihood, this model can be used in clinical applications that can reduce the necessity of in-laboratory nocturnal sleep studies since it has surpassed current classification approaches in terms of accuracy, simplicity, cost, time efficiency, and generalization. The correlation between snoring and AH1 was evaluated, though there was no measurement of vasopressin-positive and vasoactive-intestinal-polypeptide (AVP) neurons in postmortem examination of suprachiasmatic nucleus (SCN), as there was no death case. To the contrary, focus was set on the analysis of sleep disturbances that could be interpreted as the result of altered SCN function. The relationship between Snoring and AHI for the elderly with regard to its clue and impact on INSOMNIA is presented. The relationship between clinical sleep apnea and the physiological events surrounding the octogenarians was assessed. Clinically no indication for any brain tissue biopsy.

Keywords: apnea/hypopnea index (AHI), insomnia, obstructive sleep apnea, polysomnography (PSG), snoring, suprachiasmatic nucleus (SCN) nucleus, vasoactive-intestinal-polypeptide (AVP) neurons

1. Introduction

Sleep apnea is a condition that causes breathing to stop and start repeatedly during sleep. It can leave a person extremely exhausted and sleepy during the day; it is even

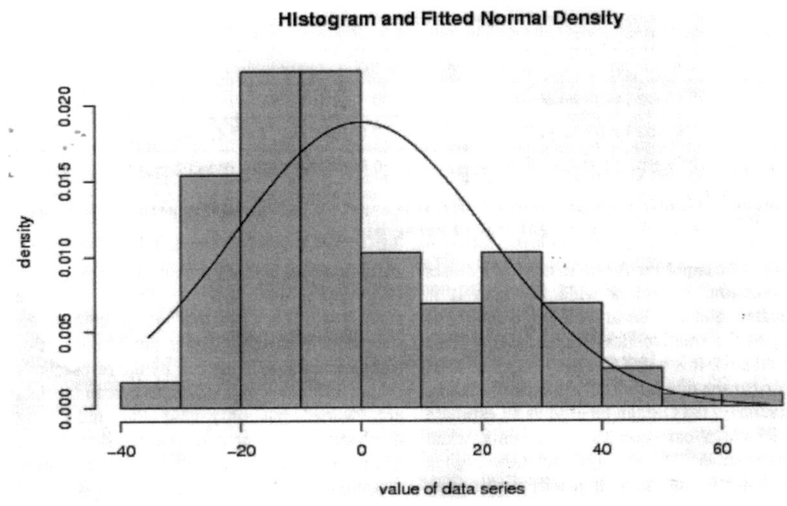

Figure 1.
Histogram of AHI distribution.

dangerous to one's own health. On the other hand, obstructive sleep apnea is the most common type of sleep apnea and it happens when the potential patients' airway is blocked and causes pauses in breathing and subsequently loud snoring. Normal snoring usually does not interfere with the quality of sleep almost as much as sleep apnea does. The author's data set were checked for normality of AHI distributions using the Kolmogorov-Smirnov's and Shapiro-Wilk's tests. The results (**Figure 1**) suggest that the data significantly deviate from a normal distribution, therefore, The null hypothesis of a normal distribution is rejected in this data set [1].

2. Materials and methods

2.1 Data collection

This study utilized the sequential collection of nocturnal EEG data from a community dwelling of older adults.

It was conducted from January 1, 2002 to January 31, 2003 at the Sleep Medicine Center (Laboratory) of Changhua Christian Hospital, Taiwan. Subjects with heart failure and chronic obstructive lung disease were excluded from the study, since there was no physician at night in the Sleep Medicine Laboratory.

The Hospital Internal Research Board and Ethical Committee approved the study, which was in conformity with the Declaration of Helsinki. The author reports no conflict of interest. Under these circumstances, among the consecutive subjects who underwent nocturnal polysomnography (PSG) during that period, there were alltogether 1,087 cases of PSG performed. The data belonged to individuals who were younger than 65 years were excluded. Hence, the inclusion criteria were (1) the chief complaint of sleep disturbance and (2) aged 65 years and over.

Therefore, 124 participants were selected out of 1,087 cases of PSG taken during study period. Not one of the participants was demented and they aged from 65 to 88.5 years. Also, no pairs of individuals were related to each other. Body mass index (BM1) data were available from 117 individuals and there were 11 octogenarians. The participants of this study provided consents that also include their personal and medical data. In addition, at the time of their initial evaluation and enrollment, they all authorized clinical data in the research database to be used in this study. All data used in accordance with the spirit and principles of Health Insurance Portability and Accountability Act regulations (H1PAA, 1996) [2]. All other data referred from other published studies with all their sources were respectively specified for the purpose of comparison. The Author reports no conflict of interest. Each individual gave a written informed consent. This author reports no conflict of interest.

2.2 Apnea hypopnea index

Initially, the subjects accomplished the Epworth Sleepiness Scale and Quality of Life SF-36 (QOL) sleep questionnaires to measure excessive daytime sleepiness (ESG). This tool is widely recognized and accepted because it is simple to use. The results of polysomnography (PSG) were collected from the participants and evaluated based on the apnea hypopnea index (AH1). There was a significant reduction in QOL for the apneic subjects. The degree of reduction was proportional to severity. For apneics with AH1 >30, there was greater impact on vitality, physical functioning, social functioning, mental health, and emotional functioning. Among the total 124 individuals, there was no single one who was demented. There was no pair of individuals related to each other.

2.3 Obstructive sleep apnea

The sleep recordings were scored according to the classification developed by Rechtschaffen and Kales [1, 3]. Kales et al used special techniques that allow subject mobility and obtain continuous electroencephalographic recordings of sleepwalkers [4]. An apneic event was defined as a reduction in airflow greater than ≥ 90% for a duration of 10 seconds or longer. A hypopneic event was scored if there is a decrease of airflow for at least 10 seconds in respirations, a 30-percent reduction in ventilation, and a decrease in oxygen saturation. The apnea hypopnea index (AH1) was calculated as the sum of events of apneas and hypopnea as per hours of nocturnal sleep. Subject with an AH1 of five or more was considered as having a diagnosable case of obstructive sleep apnea (OSA).

2.4 Polysomnography

Polysomnography (PSG) was conducted from 9:30 pm to 6:30 am in the sleep laboratory using Alice 4 Sleep Diagnostic System, Respironics, Carlsbad, Calif, USA and finger pulse oxymetry (model N 200. Nellcor, Hayward, California, U. S.). As far as the recordings are concerned, the latter included recording the central and occipital electroencephalogram (EEG) derivations (C3, C4, Ol, O2), bilateral electrooculogram (left outer canthus and right outer canthus), submental and anterior tibialis electromyogram (EMG), electrocardiogram, nasal/oral airflow were using a thermistor, respiratory effort using chest and abdominal inductance belts.

2.5 Sleep-disordered breathing

Sleep-disordered breathing (SDB) has been defined as having AH1 score of five or higher.

3. Results

3.1 Data analysis

The variables used in the analysis of the studied data contain some missing height data. Consequently, there is same small amount of missing BMI data, with less than 5.64 % (7/124) of the sample. Conversely, as compared with another data of 1,014 (aged 65 and over) control subjects came from 15,798 subjects who had participated in the Nutrition and Health Survey in Taiwan (NSC 93WFD2000205), between 1993 and 1996, one can tell that a missing rate of 5.64% is rather small. Age and blood pressure of those 1,014 subjects were analyzed and there were 665 subjects with complete data of their age, blood pressure, weight, height, and BMI, while 95.79% (15,133/15,798) of the control subjects were missing one or more of the above listed information. AH1 is classified according to the following 4 classes: < 5, between 5-15, between 15 and 30, and those > 30. For those AH1 equate and greater than 15, t test was done, and its p value is 0.023, which is significant. An independent t test was done to compare snorers and non-snorers who had AH1 at least 15, the result shows that there is a significant difference with a p value $= 0.023$. The point-biserial correlation coefficient which is used to measure the strength and direction of the association between one continuous variable and one dichotomous variable. It is symbolized here as rpb and pertains to the case that were collected where the variable of snoring is dichotomous and the other variable, AH1, is non-dichotomous. The dichotomous variable is treated as the X variable, its two possible values being coded as X=0 and X=l; and the non dichotomous variable, AH1 is treated as the Y variable (rpb = 0.39, two tailed $p < 0001$). On the other hand, the Spearman rank correlation coefficient between AHI and snoring, now as the continuous variable, reveals that there is a correlation coefficient rs = 0.26, with a confidential interval (Cl) of 0.09-0.42, and two tailed $p = 0.0035$. There is no inconsistency here: rpb and rs would tend to provide different measures of correlation because they are measuring correlation independently.

However, from the graph of Spearman's Rank Correlation test between AHI (RD1/T) and Snoring, it appears to be heteroskedastic, would tend to have the effect of artificially inflating the value of rpb. Among the 124 subjects of this study with sleep disturbance in this author's original study, there were 60 insomniacs. There are other related studies in 'super-healthy' elderly also independently found reduced amplitude of circadian output, whether from melatonin secretion or the ability to stay awake in the evening or stay asleep at the end of the night.

Both research teams, actually independently approximate the changes in the sleep homeostat with physiological measurements. Both involve in circadian rhythm reduction in amplitude phase. Both apply the same concept that the suprachiasmatic nucleus (SCN) declines with age, and more diminished with advanced age. Both independently follow the theory that there is a marked decrease in the total number of arginine vasopressin-positive (AVP), and vasoactive-intestinal-polypeptide neurons, and a diminishing in the suprachiasmatic (SCN) nucleus volume in 80- to 100-year-old individuals. SCN decreases in normal aging, which changes the circadian rhythms.

Those other studies independently investigate physiological mechanisms and clues resulting in diminishing SCN function, while this author's study focuses on physiological measurement of sleep disturbance and its fragmentation that could be interpreted because of altered SCN function. Obviously, sleep disturbances with the related sleep fragmentation are in the forefront to be linked by old age.

3.2 A novel finding of AHI: a quantile-quantile plots (q-q plots)

The quantile-quantile (q-q) plot is a graphical technique for determining if two data sets come from populations with a common distribution. The quantile-quantile plots of AHI suggest how far it deviates from being normal; the result is supported with kurtosis and skewness that are greater, / less than a -2 to +2 range when their standard deviations are considered. This implies that the assumption of normality appears to be not met; however, none of the measures of kurtosis and skewness on multiple linear regressions of AHI are being significant or worrisome.

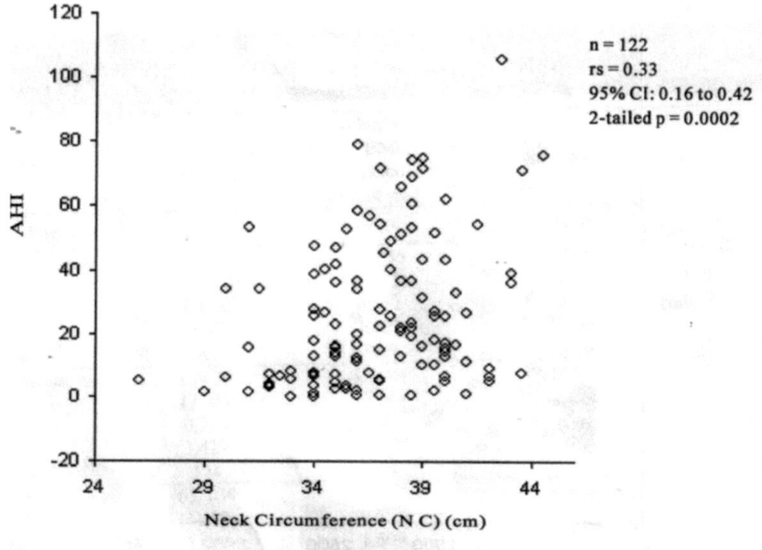

Figure 2.
The Spearman rank correlation coefficient between AHI and neck circumference.

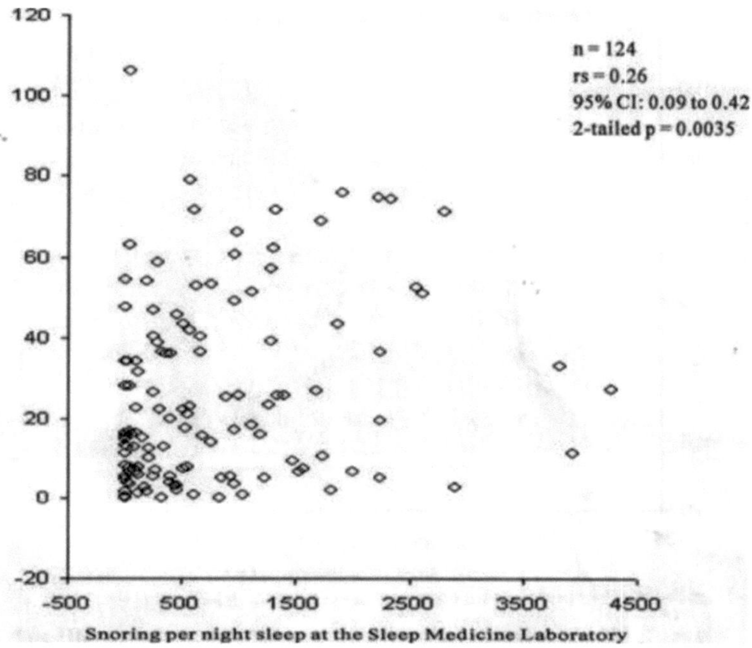

Figure 3.
The Spearman rank correlation coefficient between AHI and snoring.

3.3 AHI and BMI

BMI was calculated as weight (kilograms) divided by height squared (meters squared). It has direct relationship to obstructive sleep apnea. The upper limit of normal BMI in Far- East Asian is 23.5 kg/m2 from current WHO data. From the same set of data from one of Taiwanese studies [4–8], using the Spearman's rank correlation coefficient (rs), the correlation between AHI and BMI is 0.295 with a confidential interval (CI) of 0.09-0.42 (**Figure 2**). This rs is close to 0.330 which is the rs between AHI and neck circumstance. Therefore, the relationship between AHI and Neck Circumference can be used to approximate with that between AHI and BMI.

3.4 AHI and snoring

The Taiwanese study [5] is able to disclose that the AHI mode was 9.4 per hour; its count for 40 subjects. The highest number of AHI was 106 per hour in that study. There appears at least some effect on frequency of snoring by grouping factor of AHI. Spearman's rank correlation coefficient (rs) test revealed a mildly positive correlation between AHI and snoring (rs was 0.26) (**Figure 3**).

4. Discussion

Insomnia has been frequently caused by Sleep-disordered breathing. Sleep-disordered breathing (SDB) is defined as having AHI score of five or higher. It was 9 percent for women and 24 percent for men. According to US study, obesity, and male sex were strongly associated with the presence of sleep-disordered breathing [9]. It is important to recognize the signs and symptoms of sleep apnea, namely excessive daytime sleepiness and snoring. Prompt treatment of an underlying sleep disorder, such as OSAS, can relieve symptoms of psychiatric disease such as depression.

4.1 AHI values

A high percentage of over-65-years subjects have AHI > 5 in the US. Not all elders need to be all treated only if their AHIs are greater than five are, including but not limited to those degree 1 of Severity in our current studied subjects. An AH1 > 5 have conventionally been a cutoff point for the existence of SDB. A relatively higher point of cut-off of AHI > 15 has been used, especially for the elderly, in most of sleep studies. Those that have an AHI > 20 require treatment. Without treatment, obstructive sleep apnea can lead to serious complications and may lead to several life-threatening conditions. The responses to any treatment at different levels of AHI have received scant research attention, therefore, it is unclear that AHI is a risk factor for those aged over 65 years. However, a report in English by Ancoli-Israel et al [10] presented that it was central sleep apnea that is largely a risk factor and not obstructive apnea. Central sleep apnea occurs when the brain does not send proper signals to the muscles that control breathing. Therefore, central apnea predicts mortality above age of 65 years; others also published almost similar data [5, 11].

4.2 AHI and age

There are some other published studies that reported there is a marked decrease in the total number of AVP and vasoactive-intestinal-polypeptide neurons, as well as the SCN volume decreases in 80- to 100-year-old people compared with that are found in the younger normal adults. To analyze sleep disturbance as the result of altered SCN function, the age range of the sample in this study is within the assortment of 80 to 100 years of age. Attentions have been paid not only to Arginine Vasopressin-Positive (AVP) but as well to vasoactive- intestinal-polypeptide neurons, along with SCN regarding its volume and its number of neurons. With this regard, the study had 11 among the total 124 individuals being octogenarian and over, the finding will be compared with other studies [12].

In comparison, the aforementioned studies as well as the current study both independently approximate the changes in sleep homeostat with physiological measurements. Both involve in circadian rhythm reduction in amplitude phase. Both apply the same concept that the suprachiasmatic nucleus (SCN) declines with age, and more diminished with advanced age. Both independently follow the theory that there is a marked decrease in the total number of vasoactive-intestinal-polypeptide neurons, and a diminishing in the suprachiasmatic (SCN) nucleus volume in 80- to 100-year-old individuals. SCN decreases in normal aging, which changes the circadian rhythms.

Those other studies, just like this study, independently investigate physiological mechanisms and clues resulting in diminishing SCN function, while the current study focuses on physiological measurement of sleep disturbance and its fragmentation that could be interpreted because of altered SCN function. Obviously, sleep disturbances with the related sleep fragmentation, which in turn, results in INSOMNIA, are in forefront to be linked by old age (**Figure 4**).

4.3 The estimated prevalence of sleep-disordered breathing

It is known that the estimated prevalence of sleep-disordered breathing defined as an AH1 score of five or higher, was 9 percent for women and 24 percent for men. Male sex and obesity were strongly associated with the presence of sleep-disordered breathing (SDB). Conversely, habitual snorers, both men and women, tend to have a higher prevalence of AH1 of 15 or higher.

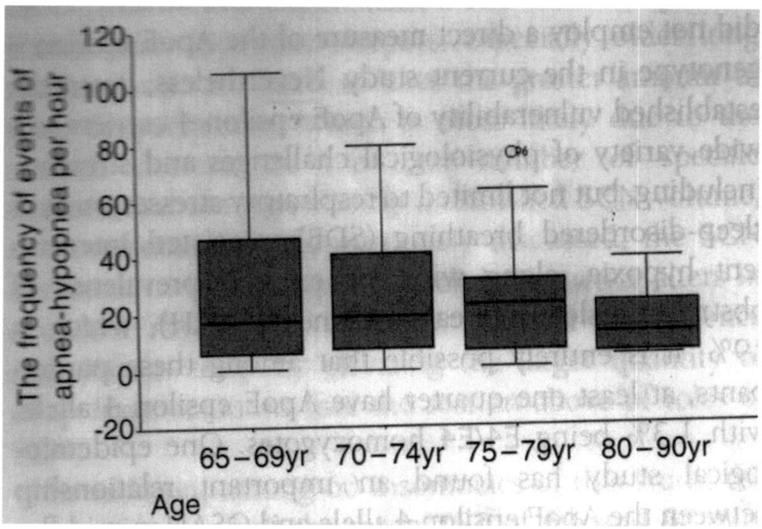

Figure 4.
Among participants who were aged 80 years and above, the minimal apnea/hypopnea index (AHI) was highest among all the age groups, while the median and maximum AHI were both lowest among all the age groups.

4.4 Difference in the two different ASSM criteria

As per the American Society of Sleep Medicine (ASSM) criteria for 1999 and 2007 respectively, it may differ on the oxyhemoglobin saturation study, but definitely, there is no difference in the sleep apnea criteria for the AHI cutoff of moderate obstructive sleep apnea. For those items that are different from both year criteria, for example, the recommended hypopnea definition of 2007, have to be met at least for the criteria as follows. The nasal pressure signal excursions decline by at least 30% of baseline. The duration of this diminishing, take place for a period lasting 10 seconds. There is an at least 4% desaturation for pre-event baseline. In addition, minimally, 90% of the event's duration must meet the amplitude reduction of criteria for hypopnea.

In addition, the difference between AASM's 1999 and 2007 in the definition of the respiratory events with regard to the severity of degree of obstructive sleep apnea is obviously identical with each other. In fact, the degrees of Sleep Apnea severity was AF11> 15/hr and > 30/hr representing respectively moderate and severe OSA according to the above criteria [13, 14]. With regard to the roles and function of the SCN, it has been clearly presented with the tabulation.

4.5 Maximum and minimum BMI

Females had mean height, weight, and cervical circumference less than the male counterparts. The female subjects had a mean BMI of 26.550 kg/m2, while male 25.19. The mean BMI of total 124 subjects was 25.574 + 4.521 kgs/m2, while that of control was 23.768 + 3.662 kg/m2, the difference was significant (the p-value < 0.0009). The Pearson's correlation coefficient between height and BMI was significantly different between males (-0.227) and females (-0.0854). In these data, the female subjects were about one year older than the male in the average. However, the female subjects had average (mean) height, weight, and cervical circumference, which were respectively less than the counter parts of the males. The 95% confidential interval for mean BM1 was 24.746-26.402. The minimum BM1 was 15.20, and maximum was 39.15.

4.6 Snoring and BMI

AH1 was noted to be correlated with BM1, snoring, body height and weight, and cervical circumference respectively. There was a highly significant correlation between BM1 and snoring. The subjects whose BMIs were more than 25 had more frequent snoring than those whose BMIs were less than 25 in the studied population. BM1 of patients was higher than control subjects. There were significant positive correlation between AH1 and BMI; Spearman's rank correlation test revealed that the relationship between snoring and BMI was highly significant.

4.7 The effect of BMI grouping on the frequency of snoring in a Taiwanese study

BMIs were classified as following three groups; group 1 (BMI > 30), group 2 (BMI between 25 and 30), and group 3 (BMI < 25). Mann-Whitney test reveals as follows. The two groups of BMI were selected for comparison. Group difference between group 1 and group 2 was insignificant (Grouping factor BMI: Mann-Whitney test, degree of freedom (d.f.) = 1, p = 0.432). Group differences either between group 1 and group 3, or group 2 and group 3 were significant (Grouping factor BMI: Mann- Whitney test, d.f. = 1, p < 0.001, p= 0.001, respectively) [5]. The groups of subjects with their BMI > 30, and a BMI between 25 and 30 snored more frequent than those in the group with a BMI < 25.

4.8 A discussion on Asian OSA prevalence

There is little information on the prevalence and severity of obstructive sleep apnea in Asian snorers although OSA may not be uncommon in Asian patients. Nevertheless, there is a single report on Singapore population that is predominantly Chinese [15]. The authors maintain that the sleep apnea syndrome is more common than the 2-4% prevalence that is quoted frequently [9]. From the snorers aged from 30-60 years in an adult population in Singapore, the authors evaluate how many snorers suffer from pathological apnea as well as sleep apnea syndrome. Within a similar age group in the same population studied with PSG in their sleep laboratory, there were 106 consecutive habitual loud snorers. The authors have found that 24.1% were loud habitual snorers. 87.5% of loud habitual snorers had significant OSA on PSG and 72% of these apneics complained of excessive daytime sleepiness (EDS). Based on the assumption that all apneics snored, the authors speculate that sleep apnea syndrome affects about 15% of the population by extrapolating these figures. EDS in their cases were validated with clinical hypersomnia [16].

There are four stages of sleep; one for rapid eye movement (REM) sleep and three that form non-REM (NREM) sleep. Less than half of brain waves consist of delta waves during stage 3 while more than half of brain activity consists of delta waves during REM sleep. Poor delta wave sleep is obviously related to hypersomnolence. OSA occurred mainly in stage 1 and 2 non-rapid eye movement (NREM) sleep instead of in REM sleep. Frequently, the arousals prevented sleep from going beyond stage 1 and 2. Because the prevalence of sleep apnea syndrome in Singaporean population aged 30-60 years exceeds one's expectations, therefore, it is likely that the people in that population, aged 30 to 60 years, suffer more hypersomnolence, which is associated with the repression of delta wave sleep by apnea occurring taking place mostly in stage 1 and 2 NREM sleep [15]. Conversely, the reported prevalence of OSA reveals as follows. The 19% of 1,775 subjects with a mean age of 71 years, SD 10.5, range 40-100 had OSA [6]. In the Philippines and Taiwan, there is no such above study.

Sleep-disordered breathing (SDB) is defined as having AH1 score of five or higher, it was 9 percent for women and 24 percent for men. According to a US study, obesity was strongly associated with the presence of sleep-disordered breathing in men [17]. In the US, a large percentage of over-65- years subjects have AH1 > 5 and elders do not need to be treated if their AHIs are greater than 5. An AHI > 5 have conventionally been a cutoff for the presence of SDB but in most of sleep studies, a higher cut-off of AHI > 15 have been used. An AHI > 20 might be better to distinguish those requiring treatment. There are not enough proposed studies that will shed light on the treatment responses at different levels of AHI. It is unclear that AHI is a risk factor for those aged over 65 years. Also, Asian's smaller upper airway merits attention. With respect to the risk factors for SDB, for example, it was reported from Singapore that other population also reported largely similar risk factors associated with habitual snoring and SDB [15]. Therefore, differential risks may highlight the importance of ethnicity in determining the burden of SDB. It is important for the health care development and research on SDB in Asia to remain alert of this circumstance in both lay and professional communities [18].

4.9 Risk factors of snoring

Snoring has independent and significant risk factor. It raises the risk for diabetes, obesity, hypertension, stroke, heart attack, and other cardiovascular problems. Snoring can create major relationship problems too. For all practical purpose, individuals were referred to the Sleep Studies because of their mixed sleep problems. It is common that an individual is unaware of his own snoring. It is not a correct assumption that subjects who did not give an account of snoring and sleepiness do not have OSA. We should always be ready to lend a hand by questioning the respective bedroom partner of a potential patient with chronic sleepiness and fatigue, or other type of sleep disturbances.

4.10 Studies on snoring

For examples, some other U S studies reveal that Tractenberg et al's findings [19, 20] were as follows. The large sample of their own 2005 and 2006 articles are originally derived from the community and they are not from a single sample with sleep disturbances. Their data still may be useful as an external and independent reference for the samples cited in this study. Hence, by comparing studies for what has been reported in this chapter, Tractenberg et al have obvious advantages on their data intake to a certain extent. This is true only if we are aggressively tracing data that have been achieved 29 years ago, for instance, as of September 2002 [19, 20]. In their studies, the criteria of the frequency of snoring were defined as: 0. for never; 1, for less than once per month; 2, for at least once per month; 3, at least, once per week; and finally, 4, nearly everyday per day/ night. Those participants who were non-demented elderly people had the frequency rating of heavily snoring from 0.7 +1.1 to 0.9 + 1.2. Those reports encounter the issue of the level of awareness of the sleep disturbance problems in the reporters at nights.

The literature estimates the prevalence habitual snoring in general population ranges from 3.6% to 35.7% [9, 21, 22]. In one of the studies in Taiwan [5], it interviewed 1,252 subjects of a sleep-medicine-laboratory based cohorts, who lived in the dwelling communities of Changhua area, Mid- Taiwan, which is adjacent to Taichung area. Their ages range from 10 to older than 60 years. 606 were males and 646 were females. The snoring prevalence in Taichung area, Taiwan, is 47.8 % for males, whereas 37.2% for females according to a report by Liu and Liu [23].

Sawit [24] has extensively reported that snoring is a risk factor for stroke, myocardial infarction, as well as acute vascular disease. In addition, habitual snorers are generally more at risk than occasional snorers. Except one by Liu and Liu [23], Taiwan does not have enough of such studies. Therefore, further studies to probe on the relationship of sleep apnea with snoring should have been carried out.

5. Conclusion

In short, other than the clarification for relationship between Snoring and AHI for the elderly as presented in this study, this study also successfully examined the relationship between clinical sleep apnea resulting in insomnia, as well as the physiological events surrounding the octogenarians among the elderly individuals studied.

Other than what has been discussed and mentioned previously, is there any model that we may follow accordingly? Certainly, there is. About twelve years ago, this author together with Yan proudly published an article entitled "A NOVEL MODEL USING GENERALIZED REGRESSION NEURAL NETWORK (GRNN) FOR ESTIMATING SLEEP APNEA INDEX IN THE ELDERLY SUFFERING FROM SLEEP DISTURBANCE. " The proposed model has sensitivity and specificity of 95.7% and 50% respectively for training cases, while 88.0% and 52.9%, respectively for the testing cases [25].

Acknowledgements

With regard to the ASSM 2007 criteria on the definition of hypopnea, this author has enjoyed his communication with Chen-Liang Lin, PhD, Department of Mechanical & Electro-Medical Engineering, National Sun Yat-Sen University, Kaohsiung, Taiwan. Thanks are due to Professor Anna Wirz-Justice, President of Society for Light Treatment and Biological Rhythms, and Professor of Psychiatry, University of Basel, Switzerland, for her courtesy and cooperation in exchanging research experiences with this author. Thanks are also due to Dr Yemeng Chen, President of New York College of Traditional Chinese, Medicine, Mineola, New York, USA. Dr So-Jen, Kuo, President of Changhua Christian Medical Center,Taiwan, and, Professor Sui- Tien Chen, Director of Systemic Biological Laboratory, Institute of Biological Chemistry, Academia Sinica, Taiwan for their respective encouragements. The author, (B. Tang) has been so grateful to his eldest son. Jack Tang, B.S. for his technical support.

Author details

Bing Tang[1,2]

1 Research and Ethics, Danville, California, USA

2 Systemic Biological Laboratory Institute of Biological Chemistry Academia Sinica, Taipei, Taiwan

*Address all correspondence to: prof.bing@gmail.com

References

[1] Jacobson A, Kales A, Lehmann D, Zweizig Jr. Somnambulism: All-Night Electroencephalographic Studies. Science. 1965 May 14;148(3672):975-7

[2] U.S. Department of Health and Human Services. Health insurance portability and accountability act of 1996. Public Law. 1996; 140-91.

[3] Rechtschaffen A. Wolpert EA, Dement WC, et al. Nocturnal sleep of narcoleptics. Electroencephalorgr Clin Neurophysiol. 1963; 15:599-609.

[4] Tang, B. A comparison study on senior sleep apnea with biostatistical and biomedical evaluations Med J Southern Taiwan 2008; 4: 73-90.

[5] Tang, B. Living by a biological clock: Age-related functional changes of sleep homeostasis in people aged 65-88.5 years. Sleep Biol Rhythms 2007; 5: 180-95.

[6] Tang, B. The correlation between snoring and apnea/ hypopnea index in the elderly, along with the Octogenarians' comparison study. Med J Southern Taiwan 2009; 5: 66-74.

[7] Tang, B. Roles of apolipoprotein-e4, and suprachiasmatic nucleus: Age related cognitive decline and sleep disordered breathing/ sleep fragmentation. In Vivo 2008; 30: 10-8.

[8] Tang, B. A comment on predicting continuous positive airway pressure from a modified split-night protocol in moderate to severe obstructive sleep apnea-hypopnea syndrome. Intern Med 2009; 48: 1489.

[9] Young, T., Palta., M, Dempsey., J, et al.The occurrence of sleep-disordered breathing among middle-aged adults. N Engl J Med 1993; 328: 1230- 5.

[10] Ancoli-Israel, S., Engler, R. L., Friedman, P. J., et al. Comparison of patients with central sleep apnea: With and without Cheyne-Stokes respiration. Chest 1994;106: 780-6.

[11] Lavie, L. and Lavie, P. Elevated plasma homocysteine in older shift-workers: A potential risk factor for cardiovascular morbidity. Chronobiol Int 2007; 24: 115-28.

[12] Hofman MA, Swaab DF. Living by the clock: the circadian pacemaker in older people. Ageing Res Rev. 2006; 5: 33-51.

[13] Sleep-related breathing disorders in adults: recommendations for syndrome definition and measurement techniques in clinical research: the report of an American Academy of Sleep Medicine Task Force. Sleep. 1999; 22: 667-689.

[14] Collop NA, Anderson WM, Boehlecke B,et al. American Academy of Sleep Medicine Clinical guidelines for the use of unattended portable monitors in the diagnosis of OS A in adult patients. Portable Monitoring Task Force of the American Academy of Sleep Medicine. J Clin Sleep Med. 2007; 15; 3:737-747.

[15] Puvanendran, K., Goh, K. L. From snoring to sleep apnea in a Singapore population. Sleep Res Online 1999; 2: 11-4.

[16] Tang, b. The impact of cultural changes on the relationship between Senior sleep disturbance and body mass index among older Adults in two asian societies. melatonin, sleep and insomia. 2009 ed. By yolanda e. Soriento. 161-189.

[17] American Academy of Sleep Medicine Task Force. Sleep-related breathing disorders in adults: Recommendations for syndrome definition and measurement techniques in clinical research: The report of an

American Academy of Sleep Medicine Task Force. Sleep 1999; 22: 667-89.

[18] Lam, B., Lam, D. C., Ip, M. S. Obstructive sleep apnoea in Asia. Int J Tuberc Lung Dis 2007; 11:2-11.

[19] Tractenberg RE, Singer CM, Cummings JL,et al. The sleep disorders inventory: An instrument for studies of sleep disturbance in persons with Alzheimer's disease. J Sleep Res 2003; 12: 33 1-7.

[20] Tractenberg RE, Singer CM, Kaye JA. Characterizing sleep problems in persons with Alzheimer's disease and normal elderly. J Sleep Res 2006;15: 97-103.

[21] Rice, D. H., Persky, M. Snoring: Clinical implications and treatment. Otolaryngol Head Neck Surg 1986; 95: 28-30.

[22] Koskenvuo, M., Kaprio, J., Partinen, M., et al. Snoring as a risk factor for hypertension and angina pectoris. Lancet 1985; 1: 893-6.

[23] Liu, S. A., Liu, H. Y. Prevalence of snoring in Taichung area: An epidemiological study. J Chin Med Assoc 2004; 67: 32-6.

[24] Sawit, S., Cabildo, J. E. S, Roxas, AA Jr. Snoring as a risk factor for stroke and myocardial infarction. Philipp J Intern Med 2006; 44: 117-24.

[25] Tang, b., Yan w. A novel model using generalized regression neural network (grnn) for estimating sleep apnea index in the elderly suffering from sleep disturbance. melatonin, sleep and insomnia. 2009 ed. By yolanda e. Soriento. 191-203.

Chapter 6

Elements of Diagnosis and Non-surgical Treatment of Obstructive Sleep Apnea in Adults from the Dental Medicine Perspective

Teodor Trăistaru, Mihaela Pantea,
Ana Maria Cristina Țâncu and Marina Imre

Abstract

Dentists hold a key role in the context of ever-growing concerns regarding the management of Obstructive Sleep Apnea (OSA) in adults. Dentists' contribution in this domain starts with the screening of patients with possible OSA. An earlier intervention for correcting a dento-maxillary anomaly or a parafunction will often serve as a preventive treatment with regard to possible OSA. Furthermore, dental medicine offers nowadays, apart from orthodontic and surgical treatment, a set of therapeutical methods, the most commonly used being the oral appliance and myofunctional therapies. Another important sphere of professional responsibility of the dentist involved in the treatment of OSA consists of periodical examinations focused on assessing clinical evolution, corrective interventions on oral appliances and interventions for preventing local complications. On the other hand, recent studies indicate the potential of different pharmacotherapy agents on OSA pathophysiology, severity and treatment. These agents have shown promising results in improving the efficacy of other therapies dedicated to OSA, therefore, current topics in modern scientific research include the evaluation of standard, even higher doses of single agents or the combination of different agents on the evolution of OSA, as well as the assessment of the association of diverse pharmacotherapy agents with other OSA therapies.

Keywords: Obstructive Sleep Apnea, Dental Sleep Medicine, Oral Appliances, Myofunctional Therapy, Pharmacotherapy Agents

1. Introduction

Sleep disorders represent an increasingly common pathology, whose undesirable effects could profoundly affect patients' every-day life. The sleep-related breathing disorders (SRBD) are placed by the American Academy of Sleep Medicine (AASM) among the six categories of sleep disorders in the International Classification of Sleep Disorders, Third Edition (ICSD-3) [1–3]: insomnia; sleep-related breathing disorders; central disorders of hypersomnolence; circadian rhythm sleep–wake disorders; parasomnias; sleep-related movement disorders. Moreover, seep-related breathing disorders - that are characterized by abnormalities of respiration during sleep - are classifies into four major categories: OSA (obstructive sleep apnea); CSA (central sleep apnea); sleep-related hypoventilation disorders; sleep-related hypoxemia disorder [4].

Obstructive Sleep Apnea (OSA) in adults represent a pathology included in the SRBD, which is associated with repetitive episodes of partial or complete collapse of the upper airway during sleep. As a result of these episodes, reduced (hypopnea) or absent (apnea) airflow lasting for at least 10 seconds is registered [3, 4]. In this specific context, the blood oxygen saturation is reduced and the brain is therefore alarmed, so "micro arousals" ("cortical arousal") appear during sleeping. Apnea episodes can repeat hundreds of times a night, without the patient being aware of them. However, the sleep-quality becomes poor, physiological sleep-pattern is disturbed and the individuals are constantly tired during the day, their work performance is affected and their quality of life decreases; moreover, individuals can even cause various work, road or domestic accidents due to excessive day-time sleepiness. OSA is a potentially life-threatening disease, its consequences including high blood pressure, diabetes, heart attack or stroke [3–5].

Obstructive sleep apnea (OSA) is traditionally quantified initially with testing during sleep by the apnea-hypopnea index (AHI), respiratory disturbance index (RDI) or respiratory event index (REI) [1, 4]. AHI results after analyzing a polysomnography (PSG) that is usually done in a sleep laboratory, and includes total episodes of apneas and total hypopneas per hour of sleep. RDI represents the sum of total apneas, total hypopneas and respiratory efforts related to arousals per hour of sleep. REI is a measure of respiratory events in a certain sleep unit of time, when using a home sleep apnea testing (HSAT); it is estimated that REI can underestimate the real index of respiratory events and OSA severity. However, the diagnosis of OSA is frequently based on the combination of clinical assessment and a diagnostic sleep study (an in-laboratory polysomnography/PSG or a home sleep study) [6].

OSA evidence-based therapeutic options includes: medical, surgical, behavioral strategies and adjuvant therapy/pharmacotherapy agents. Medical therapy is represented by PAP - positive airway pressure - therapy (CPAP/continuous positive airway pressure - the device deliver a steady pressure rate for both inhalation and exhalation); BPAP/bilevel positive airway pressure - the device deliver different pressure rates for inhalation and exhalation); APAP/automatic positive airway pressure - automatically adjusts to meet each specific person's night breathing needs) and oral appliances therapy (OAT), which aim is to reposition intraoral or craniofacial structures in order to increase the pharyngeal airway space, thus preventing pharyngeal collapse [4, 6].

Surgical options dedicated to OSA patients include: the reduction of soft tissues (i.e. adeno-tonsillectomy, uvulo-palatopharyngoplasty, tongue reduction), maxillomandibular surgery, hyoid repositioning, the increment of nasal patency [7], hypoglossal nerve stimulation (HGNS).

On the other hand, behavioral strategies are represented by the following: weight loss - ideally up to a body mass index BMI <25 kg/m^2; exercising; avoiding the consumption of tobacco and recreational substances; avoiding caffeine and alcohol before bed [1, 8]; positional therapy (non-supine position during sleep) [6, 9–12]. Different studies highlighted that weight loss is an important tool in OSA treatment, being effective in lowering OSA severity and reducing cardiovascular risks [6, 13–15].

PAP treatment is considered first-line treatment for OSA, however, its adherence is often poor [5]. The necessity for novel treatment options to help those who cannot adhere to positive airway pressure treatment is highly emerging. Regarding OAT therapy, which is enthusiastic received and applied by specialized trained dentists, several barriers were also identified, including the difficulty to accurately predict which patients will receive therapeutic benefit from this therapy and the possible side-effects related to oral appliances (OA). On the other hand, different classes of medication have been tested with regards to their effect on OSA severity. This paper will present dentists' key role in the context of ever-growing concerns regarding the management of OSA in adults, in conjunction with relevant arguments that indicate the rising potential of different pharmacotherapy agents on OSA.

2. Dentist's role in screening and treating OSAS

2.1 Identification of possible sleep disorders

In order to provide high-quality healthcare services to patients with OSAS, medical practitioners - including dentists - should adhere to the latest standards of care and should be able to participate effectively and efficiently in the management of these pathologies, according to evidence-based practices [1, 16]. Medical interdisciplinary collaboration represents a major element for diagnosis and treatment of patients with OSA. The expanding medical knowledge and the new advancements in scientific research on diverse OSA therapies place the dentist in a key-role position in the context of managing OSA in adults. Along with other medical specialists (sleep medicine specialists, pneumologists, ENT - ear, nose, and throat specialists, neurologists, cardiologists, endocrinologists, bariatric surgeons, maxillofacial surgeons, psychiatrists, psychologists), the specialists in the domain of dental sleep medicine (DSM) can participate both in the identification of possible sleep disorders and in the treatment of certain types of sleep pathologies (snoring, bruxism, mild or even moderate OSA), as well [17].

The specificity of the theoretical and practical content of dental medicine offers the practitioner of dental medicine the chance to contribute to solving medical-dental problems for a large number of patients, whose age can range from youngest to oldest. The professional and social responsibility requires that the dentist pays special attention to specific morpho-functional aspects at the level of the dento-maxillary apparatus (stomatognathic system) which, for certain patients, can suggest the presence of earlier or more advanced OSA manifestations.

Therefore, dentist's role in the management of OSA starts with the screening of the patients visiting the dental office. The screening guidelines for detection of possible sleep disorders recommend that data can be collected even from anamnesis and clinical - general and local - direct observations. The "suspect patient" with possible OSA often has a specific profile, reporting: daytime sleepiness; difficulties in daily activities; chronic fatigue; attention, concentration and memory problems; behavioral disorders: irritability, anxiety, aggressiveness; episodes of wheezing, gasping, choking, snoring or bruxism during sleep (bruxism occurs in up to 95% of patients with OSA) [3, 4]; tooth tapping; night-sweating; leg or arm movements during sleep; frequent urination during night; dry mouth sensation in the morning; morning headaches and dizziness. These elements are frequently observed: obesity; large neck-size (>43 cm for men; >40 cm for women); hypertension; gastro-esophageal reflux; age over 50; dysmenorrhea, amenorrhea, menopause; smoking; alcohol consumption [3, 4].

Along with these general aspects, dentist should notice and register local aspects that can be related to possible sleep disorders: large tonsils, voluminous posterior palatal soft tissues, hypotonic palatal or lingual musculature, tongue size (macro-glosia), tongue indentation, maxillary compression, maxillary micro-gnatism, micro-gnathism, mandibular retrognatism, deep palate, dental malposition, partial edentulous areas, tooth wear, narrow superior air-ways, oral breathing, deviated nasal septum, nose shape (narrowing) and obstructions [3, 4].

Nevertheless, patients with possible OSA will receive a thorough, complete oral examination of soft and hard tissues, and a direct examination of the temporomandibular joint (TMJ) [18]. Intraoral and extraoral photographs, full dental arch impressions for obtaining dental study casts, intraoral scanning for obtaining digital models, conventional radiological exams and additional CBCT (Cone-beam computed tomography) exams are recommended.

Application of specific questionnaires represents another important "tool" in the screening of patients with possible OSA in the dental practice; the most used questionnaires are EPWORTH and STOPBANG questionnaires [17]. Ideally, dentists should apply the questionnaires for all patients that are susceptible of OSAS. Based on data collected from anamnesis, clinical and para-clinical investigations, and on questionnaires' results, the dentists should refer the patients with possible OSA to the sleep medicine specialist.

2.2 Diagnosis and treatments of OSA: an interdisciplinary collaboration

In order to evaluate the sleep disorders, the sleep medicine specialists will perform specific clinical examinations and para-clinical tests on patients with possible sleep apnea, that were referred by the dentists (i.e. polysomnography – an overnight test that includes the monitoring of the patient's airflow through the nose and mouth; blood oxygen level/pulse-oximetry; blood pressure; electrocardiographic activity/ECG; brain wave pattern/electroencephalogram/EEG; eye movement/ Electrooculography/EOG; movement of respiratory muscle and limbs). Additionally, interdisciplinary collaboration between sleep medicine specialists and pneumologists, cardiologists, E.N.T. - ear, nose, and throat - specialists, neurologists, endocrinologists or psychiatrists is very useful for obtaining relevant data regarding the patient's general health status. The sleep medicine specialists will establish the diagnosis and severity of OSA based on previously collected data [3, 4, 16], mostly determined by the combination of clinical assessment and a diagnostic sleep study (an in-laboratory polysomnography/PSG or a home sleep study) [6].

OSA are classified as central, obstructive and combined, depending on their specific ethio-pathogenic mechanism. As previously stated, apnea-hypopnea index (AHI) is a very important element in establishing the severity of OSAS; it represents the number of times in an hour when a sleeping person either stops breathing completely or inhales limited air-flow. Each episode must last at least 10 sec. AHI is a major indicator for obstructive sleep apnea, as follows: AHI of 30 or more events in an hour indicates severe sleep apnea; AHI = 15–30 events suggests moderate apnea; AHI = 5–15 events indicates mild apnea [3, 4].

The sleep medicine specialists are responsible for establishing the proper therapy for OSA patients. The therapeutic conventional options for OSA in adults are: medical, behavioral, surgical and adjuvant - pharmacotherapy agents.

CPAP (Continuous Positive Airway Pressure) Therapy - introduced by Sullivan in 1981 - is considered the main treatment for OSA (severe, moderate and mild forms). The evaluation of the evolution of OSA under this specific therapy is assessed according to: reduction of daytime sleepiness, specific evaluation of OSA, patient and family satisfaction, adherence to therapy, achieving an optimal amount of sleep per day, practicing proper sleep hygiene, weight reduction, evaluation of factors that may aggravate the condition, titration (polysomnography/PSG) [3, 4]. CPAP therapy (Continuous Positive Airway Pressure Therapy) is frequently recommended for severe sleep apnea. On the other hand, specific recommendations are usually accepted with regard to the oral appliance therapy [1, 16, 19, 20]. Oral appliance therapy should be used only when the patient cannot endure or refuses the CPAP therapy, as some specific problems related to the use of CPAP therapy can appear: dry mouth, eye watering, chest pressure, cold sensation, frequent awakenings, noise, mask-leak, skin irritations, claustrophobia [3, 4]. Adherence to CPAP therapy (defined as > 4 h average nightly use) is considered poor with only 46–83% being adherent, even for severe and moderate OSA [3, 4, 6, 21]. Additionally, the effectiveness of oral appliances in these severe cases of OSA is estimated to be also poor. On the other hand, oral appliance therapy can be recommended as an additional treatment in the case of moderate apnea and can be the first-choice treatment in mild apnea cases. Moreover, the sleep medicine specialist who diagnoses the OSA refers the patients who could eventually benefit from OAT (oral appliance therapy) to the special trained dentist; following the complete specialized examination of the recommended patients, the dentist will decide the possibility of applying the oral appliance therapy (OAT).

2.3 Oral appliance therapy (OAT)

Oral appliance therapy (OAT), is considered - for more than 20 years - a minimally invasive and effective treatment of OSAS. Oral appliances are represented by tongue retaining devices/TRD (which hold the tongue in a more anterior position) and mandibular advancement devices/MAD (mandibular advancement appliances or mandibular repositioning appliances/MRAs) [3, 4, 6, 22]. The reviewed scientific studies highlighted that the largest evidence base and guidelines exist for mandibular advancement devices [6]. These devices include a custom-made adjustable monobloc or double occlusal splint (corresponding to the upper and lower dental arches) that has the role to anteriorly reposition the mandible and the adjacent soft tissues (including the tongue) during sleep. This stabilized position of the mandible will enable a larger opening of the pharynx lumen, which mechanically keeps the upper airway open during sleep, by preventing the soft tissue of the throat and the tongue from collapsing into the airway [17, 20, 23]. It is strongly advisable that OSA treatment should never be initiated by a dentist without the patient's assessment by a sleep medicine specialist. At this specific stage, interdisciplinary collaboration with orthodontists, specialists in prosthodontics, radiologists, specialists in geriatric dentistry, gerontologists, air-way prosthodontic specialists, TMD (temporomandibular disorders)/Oro-facial pain specialists or maxillo-facial surgeons is recommended in order to carefully prepare the sequences of the treatment plan. The results obtain via general and local examination performed by the dentists are essential not only in identifying patients with possible OSAS, but in the confirmation of the proper candidates for oral appliance therapy [18]. Moreover, the selection of the appropriate oral appliance for a specific clinical case is the responsibility of the dentists who are specialized in the treatment of sleep apnea [3, 4], and is influenced by diverse elements, as follows: characteristics of cranio-facial structures; oral condition (number, location and health-status of remaining teeth; periodontal tissues status; soft tissue health); oral functionality; anticipated dental restorative needs; reported allergies and/or sensitivities; patients' manual dexterity, visual acuity and cognitive ability; patients' comfort; financial considerations [1, 3, 4]. At the moment, more than 100 types of oral appliances are available on the medical market (i.e.: IST – Intraoral Snoring Appliance; Monoblock, Klearway; TAP-T Thornton Adjustable Positioner; Erkodent – Silensor; Somnodent; boil and bite – ready-made splints etc). A custom, titratable appliance is recommended versus a non-custom oral device [16, 19], as a successful oral appliance therapy (OAT) is considered to be an integrated, customized treatment. The oral appliances are small-sized, portable, easy to tolerate and easy to clean.

The two occlusal splints of the oral appliance are connected by a special system that allows the stabilization of the mandible in a protrusive position. 75% of the maximum protrusion of the mandible, i.e. approximately 8-9 mm on average, is usually recommended to be determined and registered for the most oral appliances; this amount of protrusion is considered to be the maximum allowed for an oral appliance therapy dedicated to OSAS. The adjustment of mandibular advancement level (titration) is recommended to be included in the specific monitoring of OSA patient (part of the immediate check-ups and long-term follow-ups, as well).

Obtaining an oral appliance involves several successive steps: conventional impressions of the dental arches or intraoral scanning; obtaining the models of the dental arches (cast models, 3D printed models or digital ones); registration of the protrusive position of the mandible; project and fabrication of the oral appliance; oral appliance delivery: intra-oral placement, control and adjustments; use and homecare instructions delivery.

Regarding the registration of the protrusive position of the mandible for OAT, findings in medical literature suggest that a 25–75% protrusion is ranged as comfortable and yet therapeutic [24, 25]. On the other hand, maximizing the mandibular protrusion with oral appliances may be more important in severe cases of apnea. Different studies highlighted that the treatment results with oral appliances are better when the mandibular advancement is greater - however, possible associated local side effects should be observed and fixed [24, 26]. The protruded mandibular position can be determined and registered with special devices (i.e. "The George Gauge™ Kit").

As stated before, patients undergoing oral appliance therapy should be informed and educated about the correct night-wear of the appliance, about its insertion, disinsertion and proper cleaning; morning exercises (using, for example, the Occlusion Trainer [18]), gymnastics and facial, head and neck massages are recommended as well [1, 19].

Nevertheless, patients should be aware of the importance of weight control and sleep hygiene; a proper lifestyle, which involves a healthy diet, gymnastics, sports, avoiding caffeine, alcohol, tobacco or recreational substances [1, 3, 4, 8] can have a positive effect on the results of oral appliances therapy. Additionally, positional therapy is considered to be a beneficial adjunct to oral appliance therapy, in order to reduce AHI across total sleep time [6, 25, 27].

Oral myofunctional therapy (OMT) is also recommended to be associated with OA therapy [4]. Suzuki et al. showed that application of OMT was accompanied with a decrease of AHI by approximately 50% in a group of students with high Epworth Sleepiness Scale (ESS) [28]. Upper airway muscle training (oropharyngeal exercises, breathing, speech, swallowing, chewing exercises, movement of the tongue, nose, cheeks, and jaw) completed for 3 months (one hour per day) could decreased the AHI by 39% in patients with moderate OSA [29].

Immediate check-ups and also long-term follow-ups are needed after the insertion of a mandibular advancement device (MAD). Appointments are made within the first days or, at least, within the first two weeks after the delivery of the oral appliance; patient comfort and the efficacy of the applied treatment should first be assessed by the dentists, along with small adjustments of the appliance that are also recommended, such as reduction of the pressure against the teeth or marginal fit adjustments. Titration/calibration of the oral appliance is a very delicate and important aspect in oral appliance therapy. Continued gradual advancement of the mandible may bring further improvement of the symptoms related to OSA [1, 3, 4, 16]. On the other hand, sometimes reduction of the mandibular protrusion is necessary, if adverse local effects are registered. The oral appliance therapy outcomes are evaluated by the sleep medicine specialists three months after the initiation of the OA treatment; a control polysomnography is recommended and the progress and benefits of the treatment should be registered.

Periodical examinations focused on assessing clinical evolution, corrective interventions on oral appliances, as well as the interventions for preventing the oro-dental complications - that oral appliances can generate - represent another sphere of professional responsibility of the dental practitioner involved in the OSA treatment. Periodical dental and medical check-ups (every six months or at least once a year) are strongly recommended for long-term monitoring of patients with OSA. The management of this patients in long term imply permanent communication between the dentists, the patient's physician and other healthcare professionals that were involved in the treatment. The dentist should check and register: patient comfort; oral appliance efficacy; persistence of previously resolved symptoms related to OSA; the structural integrity and the occlusal stability of the oral appliance; wear, fractures; bacterial or fungal growth on the appliance [1, 4]. During this periodical dental examinations the appearance of possible side effects correlated to oral appliance therapy can be observed: muscle and joint soreness; soft tissue or gingival inflammation; excessive salivation or, on the contrary, dry mouth sensation; tooth mobility or fractures; teeth migrations and occlusion disturbances [3, 4, 30]. All side effects produced by the oral appliance therapy should be registered, documented and managed; it is important to determine the possible causes of these unpleasant side-effects and to try to reduce the damage. Balance between the actual need of oral appliance therapy and the severity of generated side effects should be evaluated in order to determine if oral appliance therapy should be discontinued and if the patient agree with another form of therapy recommended by the physician. Yet, Lavigne [4] consider that the adverse effects of oral appliances are generally considered to be negligible, mild or transient among most patients.

3. Pharmacotherapy agents and OSA pathophysiology

The use of medical-dental therapies, as stand-alone or in combination with other therapeutical alternatives for controlling OSA, represent a viable option in certain clinical cases, depending on the OSA clinical severity and/or the patient's acceptance of the suggested solution. As pharmacotherapy agents have shown good results in improving the efficacy of other therapies dedicated to OSA, modern scientific research in the field of OSA focuses on the evaluation of diverse doses of single agents or the combination of different agents on the evolution of OSA. Another important aspect regards the association of diverse pharmacotherapy agents with other conventional OSA therapies.

Hypnotics represent a group of pharmacological agents that promote sleep and moderate sedation by depressing the central nervous system. Hypnotic use is relatively frequent for people diagnosed with OSA, as they usually experience current insomnia [31]. Interest has grown steadily in the current scientific research to determine the specific effects of hypnotics on OSA severity, pathophysiology, their possible side-effects.

Benzodiazepines have sedative-hypnotic, myorelaxant, and anticonvulsive actions, in higher doses being commonly prescribed for insomnia [31]; early studies suggested that their use in patients with OSA has been controversial and can possibly worsen overnight hypoxemia in OSA [32, 33].

Hoijer et al. [32] reported in 1994 that nitrazepam did not adversely influence apnea intensity or severity in patients with mild to moderate sleep apnea; the authors suggested that contraindicating benzodiazepine use in sleep apnea may be restricted to the patients with severe sleep apnea.

Late in 2011, a study conducted by Wang et al. [33], showed that mild–moderate OSA patients with higher awake central chemosensitivity have higher breathing impairment during sleep following the use of a hypnosedative - temazepam; in this context, the authors highlighted the clinical importance of phenotyping the individual OSA response to temazepam using ventilatory chemoreflexes during wakefulness.

A relatively recent study, conducted by Lin BM et al. [34] confirm that the use of benzodiazepine receptor agonists is not associated with increased odds of snoring in middle-aged and elderly women. On the other hand, the administration of certain benzodiazepine sedatives in chronic pain patients on opioids induces mild respiratory depression, which is associated with reduced severity of OSA, probably increasing the arousal threshold [35]. However, some studies reported that benzodiazepines can produce poor motor coordination, dizziness or next-day drowsiness, and can alter the cognitive process and driving ability [31].

Certain pharmacological agents used to treat depression also have sedative effects, and thus are administered to improve night-sleep. As there is an increase need to augment OSA early detection, treatment options and strategies, emerging therapies such as non-benzodiazepine sedative hypnotics (NBSH) could be considered good alternative treatments, along with weight loss, positional therapy, oral appliances, or surgery [6]. Subjects with OSA usually demonstrate a low arousal threshold or propensity to wake easily in response to a disturbance. Sedatives were tried as a therapy for OSA, and different studies highlighted that sedative agents can increase arousal threshold [6, 36–39], for example, trazodone (100 mg, taken orally, 90 min. before bedtime) - a non-myorelaxant sleep-promoting agent - increases the respiratory effort-related to arousal threshold [36] and eszopiclone (3 mg, immediately prior to sleep) also increases the arousal threshold and lowers the AHI in obstructive sleep apnea patients [38].

Recently, Chen et al. [40] studied the effect of sedative antidepressants on the severity of OSA in stroke patients, as these medication is frequently prescribed for stroke patients due to their high prevalence of depression and insomnia. Patients were administered 100 mg of trazodone (*Trazodone Tab, Taoyuan, Taiwan*) just before polysomnography. The authors reported that trazodone may decrease OSA severity without increasing nocturnal hypoxia in OSA patients with comorbid ischemic stroke. On the other hand, it is acknowledged that trazodone - a tricyclic antidepressant - can cause severe toxicity at excessive doses [31].

Z-drugs represent a class of non-benzodiazepine agents (zolpidem, zopiclone, eszopiclone, zaleplon), with certain properties that make them more attractive: they have less adverse side effects, do not reduce deep sleep, and cause less residual daytime effects [31, 41].

The effects of zopiclone – a nonbenzodiazepine sedative – on the arousal threshold and on genioglossus muscle activity were analyzed in a group of patients with predominantly severe OSA [42]; thus, the potential effects of zopiclone on obstructive sleep apnea (OSA) severity was studied. The results of this study showed that zopiclone (7.5 mg, taken orally, immediately prior to sleep) increased the arousal threshold without reducing genioglossus muscle activity; the authors noted that these aspects may be favorable for some patients with OSA.

However, despite of these promising results of different scientific studies, Eckert et al., early in 2014, [37], pointed out that no trial or evidence has demonstrated a clear and significant improvement in severity of sleep disordered breathing when sedative therapy is applied, even in patients with a low arousal threshold.

Moreover, Carter et al. [42] stated that zopiclone may worsen hypoxemia in some patients with OSA.

Yet, the effect of non-benzodiazepine sedative hypnotics (NBSH) on continuous positive airway pressure (CPAP) adherence in patients with obstructive sleep apnea (OSA) was highlighted in a recent study [43]: the authors concluded that non-benzodiazepine sedative hypnotics administered in OSA patients may increase CPAP adherence (defined as CPAP use for >4 h/night, on >70% of nights); additionally, they noted that especially eszopiclone showed the most significant effect on CPAP adherence, however, the effect of zolpidem and zaleplon on CPAP adherence requires further investigation.

Recently, orexin antagonists have been recommended primarily for people with insomnia [31, 44]. Certain roles of orexin neuropeptides (that are produced by neurons in the lateral hypothalamus) are represented by the regulation of sleep and arousal, as well of circadian rhythms; orexin neurons are activated during wakefulness, but during sleep they are inhibited [45]. Consequently, dual orexin receptor antagonists (DORAs: almorexant, lemborexant, filorexant, suvorexant) may be considered an additional pharmaceutical option to treat insomnia in some patients [44]. For example, suvorexant showed a more balanced sleep architecture profile and greater potency than almorexant, yet, no clinically meaningful respiratory effects during sleep were observed in patients with mild or moderate OSA, receiving a single dose (40 mg) or multiple doses of suvoxerant [46]. As the influence of suvorexant in patients with severe OSA have not been profoundly studied, this medication must be used with caution and administered at lower doses in patients with OSA [44].

Along with the pharmacological agents listed and presented above, antihistamines (histamine antagonists) - that are often recommended in case of respiratory allergies - have also been used to treat mild insomnia. However, they are not associated with dependence, but tolerance can occur with their long-term use.

Additionally, Carter et al., in 2021 [31], concluded that common hypnotics can increase the respiratory arousal threshold by approximately 15–30% and have inconsistent effects on next-day alertness; however, in case of obese patients, severe OSA, higher respiratory arousal threshold, or at high doses, hypnotics can worsen overnight hypoxemia.

A stated before, different mechanisms can contribute to multifactorial OSA pathophysiology [5], including: increased collapsibility of the passive upper airway; impaired neuromuscular tone (relative hypotonia of upper airway dilator muscle/genioglossus muscle) and sympathetic neural activity; greater the loop gain; anatomic craniofacial features (increased anterior facial height, decreased pharyngeal airspace, inferiorly placed hyoid bone); high body mass index (obesity); rostral fluid shifts. This heterogenous pathogenesis can generate opportunities for therapies with diverse mechanisms of action: antihypertensive medication (acetazolamide; spironolactone), anti-inflammatory agents, antidiabetic medications, antidepressant medications or synthetic cannabinoids [5]. Moreover, Lavigne, in 2009 [3], stated that "of all the metabolic syndrome components, OSA has been most strongly linked with hypertension". Different scientific studies confirm this statement. Eskandari et al. [47], conducted a study in a group of men participants with moderate to severe OSA, which was divided in three sub-groups depending on the received treatment: acetazolamide therapy only; continuous positive airway pressure (CPAP) therapy only; acetazolamide plus CPAP therapy; the authors pointed out that a reduction in AHI was found in all three experimental groups, with the greatest reduction noted in the acetazolamide plus CPAP group. It was also demonstrated that spironolactone administered to patients with moderate–severe OSA and resistant hypertension produces a change in AHI from 36.6/hour at baseline to 14.8/hour [48]. In the same line, Fiori et al. [49], showed that spironolactone plus furosemide daily reduced AHI by 14.4%, after one week of treatment, versus sodium-restricted diet that reduced AHI by 22.3% and versus 0.8% reduction of AHI correspondent to the placebo monotherapy.

As regard of Sodium-glucose Cotransporter-2 inhibitors (SGLT-2 inhibitors), there are previous studies indicating that SGLT-2 inhibitors may reduce OSA severity. Furukawa et al. [50] found that dapagliflozin might improve moderate to severe sleep-disorders breathing in Japanese patients with obesity and type 2 diabetes mellitus (mean AHI decreased from 25/hour to 19/hour). Tang et al. [51] considered that dapagliflozin could demonstrate therapeutic value for patients with T2DM (type-2 diabetes mellitus) combined with OSA; this study highlights that dapagliflozin can significantly reduce glucose, BMI, blood pressure and AHI and improve hypoxemia during sleep, therefore, indicates that dapagliflozin has potential as an effective treatment approach for OSA.

On the other hand, limited studies have been conducted in patients with OSA in order to demonstrate reduction in AHI with synthetic cannabinoids use. Yet, recently, Taranto-Montemurro L et al. [52] showed for the first time that the combination of a norepinephrine reuptake inhibitor (atomoxetine/80 mg at bedtime) and an antimuscarinic (oxybutynin/5 mg at bedtime) clearly reduces OSA Severity (>50%); the authors suggested these results may reorient future treatment of OSA.

4. Conclusions

It is well acknowledged the complexity of OSA, its heterogeneity in terms of risk factors and consequences, pathophysiological phenotypes, clinical presentation, and comorbidity [6, 53]. We understand more and more the importance of phenotyping patients with OSA (clinical, anatomical, genetic and polysomnographic phenotyping, biomarkers assessment, life style factors evaluation) and identifying the patients that can benefit from a pharmacotherapy that targets their major predisposing factors [4, 6]. This aim implies advanced validation of the phenotyping tools and algorithms that should be used to identify the principal factors precipitating OSA in individual patients [53]. The interconnected risk factors for OSA needs to be considered in order to achieve precision medicine in OSA [4]. Pharmacotherapy agents may have an important role as monotherapy in the treatment of mild OSA, or could be used in association with other therapies in moderate-to-severe OSA, including oral appliances therapy (OAT), provided by dentists trained in dental sleep medicine (DSM). Additionally, as patient-centered care is the future, recognizing and understanding patient profound medical needs, preferences, their psychological status, expectations and beliefs [4] contribute in the successful implementation of OSA complex therapies.

Moreover, considering the interest shown in the field of TMD (temporo-mandibular disorders) and oro-facial pain for under and post-graduate students training, and given the important role of the dentist in the early detection, treatment and monitoring of patients with OSA and sleep bruxism, it is necessary that the aspects related to dental sleep medicine (DSM) should also be found in a multi- and inter-disciplinary organized form in university curricula (stand-alone disciplines, courses, practical training), this approach corresponding to the growing need for treatment of this pathology in the general population.

An important issue is the one related to the actual "dental/clinical complex symbiosis" in OSA therapy, that should lead to improved personal medical care.

The combined modern therapies for OSA (medical, surgical, behavioral strategies, pharmacotherapy agents) have to be adjusted continuously, in respect to recent scientific research, in order to deliver the best results for patients, emphasizing their quality of life in addition to medical care.

Current - Western allopathic medicine benefits from the accumulation of large fundamental biomedical knowledge, special equipment, modern materials and techniques.

Medical specializations and supra-specializations offer increased chances for therapeutic success, provided that the early diagnosis and therapeutic indication are as accurate as possible and the patient has proper, legitimate access to the health services provided by the medical staff.

The complexity of clinical cases varies between patients, and the clinical complexity of a single clinical case can evolve towards simplification or, on the contrary, towards increased complexity. The greater the complexity of a clinical case is, the greater is the need for multidisciplinary collaboration, in order to increase the accuracy of medical decisions.

In our opinion, the previous considerations are also valid in the case of OSA, whose etiopathogenic and clinical complexity requires such an approach. To meet such a requirement - that focuses on the quality of life of the patient, with his unique bio-psycho-social-cultural profile, unlikely repeatable - health care systems, along with socio-economic, cultural or political systems must act in multiple directions.

First of all, the health systems should be provided with the necessary medical personnel, having various clinical specializations; nevertheless, medical personnel should have a balanced territorial distribution and it should be open to continuous training and inter-disciplinary collaboration.

Secondly, regarding the rapidly evolving topic represented by OSA, which obviously represents an interdisciplinary chapter of human pathology, it would be interesting to organize university courses with interdisciplinary content, that are opened to all students in both medicine and dentistry. This approach can create a strong basis for future interdisciplinary clinical collaborations between post-graduates. Importantly, the medical management between the dental and clinical disciplines should be optimally and formally integrated. This aspect involves the promotion of clinical guidelines suitable for dental practitioners' use, and proper training for the next generation of dentists.

Additionally, medical dental practitioners contribution in OSA management could be found in the clinically justified concern of phenotyping OSA patients, so that each patient is recommended the best (simple or combined) therapeutic variant, adjusted to the individual etiopathogenic context and to the severity of the disease.

On the other hand, properly designed both clinical and dental research studies could contribute to better specification of the various "subsets" of patients, which could thus benefit more from the application of a proper therapeutic variant. In this context, dentistry could become more useful and more effective in the management of OSA patients and cases of "over-treatment" or cases of malpractice could thus be avoided.

The role of dentistry and the involvement of dental sleep medicine specialists in prevention, detection, treatment of mild or moderate forms of OSA, and in long term management of OSA is acknowledged. Moreover, multidisciplinary and interdisciplinary medical path allow a holistic approach of the patient, thus providing best therapeutic results.

Promising results were achieved in the field of pharmacotherapy of OSA - as stand alone or in combination with other therapies. Nevertheless, more scientific research and consistent clinical trials are needed in order to offer great perspectives for this fascinating medical domain.

Conflict of interest

The authors declare no conflict of interest.

Abbreviations

AAMS	American Academy of Sleep Medicine
AHI	Apnea-Hypopnea Index
APAP	automatic positive airway pressure
BMI	body mass index
BPAP	bilevel positive airway pressure
CBCT	cone-beam computed tomography
CPAP	continuous positive airway pressure
CSA	central sleep apnea
DORAs	dual orexin receptor antagonists
DSM	dental sleep medicine
ECG	electrocardiographic activity
EEG	electroencephalogram
ENT	ear, nose, and throat specialist/surgeon
EOG	electrooculography
ESS	Epworth Sleepiness Scale
HGNS	hypoglossal nerve stimulation
HSAT	Home Sleep Apnea Testing
IST	Intraoral Snoring Appliance
MAD	mandibular advancement devices
MRAs	mandibular repositioning appliances
NBSH	non-benzodiazepine sedative hypnotics
OA	oral appliance
OAT	oral appliance therapy
OMT	oral myofunctional therapy
OSA	obstructive sleep apnea
PAP	positive airway pressure
PSG	polysomnography/polysomnogram
RDI	Respiratory Disturbance Index
REI	Respiratory Event Index
SGLT-2 inhibitors	Sodium-glucose Cotransporter-2 inhibitors
SRBD	sleep-related breathing disorders
TAP	T Thornton Adjustable Positioner
TMD	temporo-mandibular disorders
TMJ	temporomandibular joint
TRD	tongue retaining device
T2DM	type-2 diabetes mellitus

Author details

Teodor Trăistaru[1,2], Mihaela Pantea[1,2*], Ana Maria Cristina Țâncu[1,3] and Marina Imre[1,3]

1 “Carol Davila” University of Medicine and Pharmacy, Bucharest, Romania

2 Faculty of Dental Medicine, Department of Fixed Prosthodontics and Occlusology, Bucharest, Romania

3 Faculty of Dental Medicine, Department of Complete Denture, Bucharest, Romania

*Address all correspondence to: mihaela.pantea@umfcd.ro

References

[1] Levine M, Bennett K, Cantwell M, Postol K, Schwartz D. Dental sleep medicine standards for screening, treating, and managing adults with sleep-related breathing disorders. J Dent Sleep Med. 2018; 5(3):61-68. http://dx.doi.org/10.15331/jdsm.7030

[2] Zucconi M, Ferri, R. Assessment of sleep disorders and diagnostic procedures: 1. Classification of sleep disorders. Eur Sleep Res Soc - Sleep Medicine Textbook. 2014;23:95-110. http://www.esrs.eu/

[3] Lavigne GJ, Cistulli PA, Smith MT. Sleep medicine for dentists: a practical overview. Quintessentce Publishing. 2009:29,53,56,73,88,94,126,129.

[4] Lavigne GJ, Cistulli PA, Smith MT. Sleep Medicine for Dentists: An Evidence-Based Overview. 2nd Edition, Quintessentce Publishing. 2020:6,7,22-25,31-33, 50,87,88,96,104,107.

[5] Schütz SG, Dunn A, Braley TJ, Pitt B, Shelgikar AV. New frontiers in pharmacologic obstructive sleep apnea treatment: A narrative review. Sleep Medicine Reviews, 2021:101473. https://doi.org/10.1016/j.smrv.2021.101473

[6] Sutherland K, Kairaitis K, Yee BJ, Cistulli PA. (2018). From CPAP to tailored therapy for obstructive sleep Apnoea. Multidisciplinary respiratory medicine. 2018;13(1):1-13. https://doi.org/10.1186/s40248-018-0157-0

[7] MacKay SG, Chan L. Surgical approaches to obstructive sleep apnea. Sleep Med Clin. 2016;11(3):331-341. https://doi.org/10.1016/j.jsmc.2016.04.003

[8] Simou E, Britton J, Leonardi-Bee J. Alcohol and the risk of sleep apnoea: a systematic review and meta-analysis. Sleep Medicine. 2018;42:38-46. https://doi.org/10.1016/j.sleep.2017.12.005

[9] Ravesloot MJ, van Maanen JP, Dun L, de Vries N. The undervalued potential of positional therapy in position-dependent snoring and obstructive sleep apnea-a review of the literature. Sleep Breath. 2013;17(1):39-49. https://doi.org/10.1007/s11325-012-0683-5

[10] de Vries GE, Hoekema A, Doff MH, Kerstjens HA, Meijer PM, van der Hoeven JH, et al. Usage of positional therapy in adults with obstructive sleep apnea. J Clin Sleep Med. 2015;11(2):131-137. https://doi.org/10.5664/jcsm.4458

[11] Eijsvogel MM, Ubbink R, Dekker J, Oppersma E, de Jongh FH, van der Palen J, Brusse-Keizer MG. Sleep position trainer versus tennis ball technique in positional obstructive sleep apnea syndrome. J Clin Sleep Med. 2015;11(2):139-147. https://doi.org/10.5664/jcsm.4460

[12] Ravesloot MJL, White D, Heinzer R, Oksenberg A, Pepin JL. Efficacy of the new generation of devices for positional therapy for patients with positional obstructive sleep apnea: a systematic review of the literature and meta-analysis. J Clin Sleep Med. 2017;13(6): 813-824. https://doi.org/10.5664/jcsm.6622

[13] Johansson K, Neovius M, Lagerros YT, Harlid R, Rossner S, Granath F, Hemmingsson E. Effect of a very low energy diet on moderate and severe obstructive sleep apnoea in obese men: a randomised controlled trial. BMJ. 2009;339. https://doi.org/10.1136/bmj.b4609

[14] Kajaste S, Brander PE, Telakivi T, Partinen M, Mustajoki P. A cognitive-behavioral weight reduction program in the treatment of obstructive sleep apnea syndrome with or without initial nasal CPAP: a randomized study. Sleep Med. 2004;5(2):125-131. https://doi.org/10.1016/j.sleep.2003.07.007

[15] Tuomilehto HP, Seppa JM, Partinen MM, Peltonen M, Gylling H, Tuomilehto JO, Vanninen EJ, Kokkarinen J, Sahlman JK, Martikainen T, Soini EO, Randell J, Tukiainen H, Uusitupa M. Lifestyle intervention with weight reduction: first-line treatment in mild obstructive sleep apnea. Am J Respir Crit Care Med. 2009;179(4):320-327. https://doi.org/10.1164/rccm.200805-669OC

[16] Ramar K, Dort LC, Katz SG, Lettieri CJ, Harrod CG, Thomas SM, Chervin RD. Clinical practice guideline for the treatment of obstructive sleep apnea and snoring with oral appliance therapy: an update for 2015. J Clin Sleep Med. 2015;11(7):773-827. https://doi.org/10.5664/jcsm.4858

[17] Pantea M, Imre M, Trăistaru T, Perlea P, Temelcea AN, Țâncu AMC. Practical considerations and guidelines in dental sleep medicine. Romanian Journal of Oral Rehabilitation. 2018;10:44-50; http://www.rjor.ro/practical-considerations-and-guidelines-in-dental-sleep-medicine/?lang=ro

[18] Smith MT, Wickwire EM, Grace EG, Edwards RR, Buenaver LF, Peterson S, Klick B, Haythornthwaite JA. Sleep disorders and their association with laboratory pain sensitivity in temporomandibular joint disorder. Sleep. 2009;32(6):779-790. https://doi.org/10.1093/sleep/32.6.779

[19] Rogers RR, Remmers J, Lowe AA, Cistulli PA, Prinsell J, Pantino D, Rogers MB. History of dental sleep medicine. Journal of Dental Sleep Medicine2014;1(1):67-74.

[20] Schwarting S, Huebers U, Heise M, Schlieper J, Hauschild A. Position paper on the use of mandibular advancement devices in adults with sleep-related breathing disorders. Sleep Breath. 2007;11:125-126. https://doi.org/10.1007/s11325-007-0116-z

[21] Weaver TE, Sawyer A. Management of Obstructive Sleep Apnea by Continuous Positive Airway Pressure, Oral and Maxillofacial Surgery Clinics of North America. 2009; 21(4):403-412. https://doi.org/10.1016/j.coms.2009.08.001

[22] Lazard DS, Blumen M, Levy P, Chauvin P, Fragny D, Buchet I, Chabolle F. The tongue-retaining device: efficacy and side effects in obstructive sleep apnea syndrome. J Clin Sleep Med. 2009;5(5):431-438. https://doi.org/10.5664/jcsm.27598

[23] Scherr SC, Dort LC, Almeida FR, Bennett KM, Blumenstock NT, Demko BG, Essik GK, Katz SG, McLornan PM, Phillips KS, Prehn RS, Rogers RR, Schell TG, Sheats RD, Sreshta FP. Definition of an effective oral appliance for the treatment of obstructive sleep apnea and snoring. J Dent Sleep Med. 2014;1(1):39-50. http://dx.doi.org/10.15331/jdsm.3738

[24] Aarab G, Lobbezoo F, Hamburger HL, Naeije M. Effects of an oral appliance with different mandibular protrusion positions at a constant vertical dimension on obstructive sleep apnea. Clin Oral Investig. 2010;14(3):339-345. https://doi.org/10.1007/s00784-009-0298-9

[25] Sutherland K; Vanderveken OM; Tsuda H; Marklund M; Gagnadoux F; Kushida CA; Cistulli PA. Oral appliance treatment for obstructive sleep apnea: an update. J Clin Sleep Med. 2014;10(2):215-227. https://doi.org/10.5664/jcsm.3460

[26] Walker-Engstrom ML, Ringqvist I, Vestling O, Wilhelmsson B, Tegelberg A. A prospective randomized study comparing two different degrees of mandibular advancement with a dental appliance in treatment of severe obstructive sleep apnea. Sleep Breath. 2003;7:119-130. https://doi.org/10.1007/s11325-003-0119-3

[27] Dieltjens M, Vroegop AV, Verbruggen AE, Wouters K, Willemen M, De Backer WA, Verbraecken JA, Van de Heyning PH, Braem MJ, de Vries N, Vanderveken OM. A promising concept of combination therapy for positional obstructive sleep apnea. Sleep Breath. 2015;19(2):637-644. https://doi.org/10.1007/s11325-014-1068-8

[28] Suzuki H, Watanabe A, Akihiro Y, Takao M, Ikematsu T, Kimoto S, Asano T, Kawara M. Pilot study to assess the potential of oral myofunctional therapy for improving respiration during sleep. J Prosthodont Res. 2013;57:195-199. https://doi.org/10.1016/j.jpor.2013.02.001

[29] Diaferia G, Badke L, Santos-Silva R, Bommarito S, Tufik S, Bittencourt L. Effect of speech therapy as adjunct treatment to continuous positive airway pressure on the quality of life of patients with obstructive sleep apnea. Sleep Med. 2013;14:628-635. https://doi.org/10.1016/j.sleep.2013.03.016

[30] Sheats RD, Schell TG, Blanton AO, Braga PM, Demko G, Dort LC, Farquhar D, Katz SG, Masse J-F, Rogers RR, Scherr SC, Schwartz DB, Spencer J. Management of side effects of oral appliance therapy for sleep-disordered breathing. Journal of Dental Sleep Medicine. 2017;4(4):111-125. http://dx.doi.org/10.15331/jdsm.6746

[31] Carter SG, Eckert DJ. Effects of hypnotics on obstructive sleep apnea endotypes and severity: Novel insights into pathophysiology and treatment, Sleep Medicine Reviews. 2021;58:101492, ISSN 1087-0792, https://doi.org/10.1016/j.smrv.2021.101492

[32] Hoijer U, Hedner J, Ejnell H, Grunstein R, Odelberg E, Elam . Nitrazepam in patients with sleep apnoea: a double-blind placebo-controlled study. European Respiratory Journal. 1994;7(11):2011-2015. DOI: 10.1183/09031936.94.07112011

[33] Wang D, Marshall NS, Duffin J, Yee BJ, Wong KK, Noori N, Hg SSW, Grunstein RR. Phenotyping interindividual variability in obstructive sleep apnoea response to temazepam using ventilatory chemoreflexes during wakefulness. J Sleep Res. 2011;20(4):526-532. https://doi.org/10.1111/j.1365-2869.2011.00931.x

[34] Lin BM, Hu FB, Curhan GC. Association between benzodiazepine receptor agonists and snoring among women in the nurses' Health study. J Am Med Assoc Otolaryngol Head Neck Surg. 2017;143(2):162-167. https://doi.org/10.1001/jamaoto.2016.3174

[35] Mir S, Wong J, Ryan CM, Bellingham G, Singh M, Waseem R, Eckert DJ, Chung F. Concomitant benzodiazepine and opioids decrease sleep apnoea risk in chronic pain patients. Eur Respir J Open Res. 2020;6,3. DOI: 10.1183/23120541.00093-2020

[36] Heinzer RC, White DP, Jordan AS, Lo YL, Dover L, Stevenson K, Malhotra A. Trazodone increases arousal threshold in obstructive sleep apnoea. Eur Respir J. 2008;31(6):1308-1312. https://doi.org/10.1183/09031936.00067607

[37] Eckert DJ, Malhotra A, Wellman A, White DP. Trazodone increases the respiratory arousal threshold in patients with obstructive sleep apnea and a low arousal threshold. Sleep. 2014;37(4):811-819. https://doi.org/10.5665/sleep.3596

[38] Eckert DJ, Owens RL, Kehlmann GB, Wellman A, Rahangdale S, Yim-Yeh S, et al. Eszopiclone increases the respiratory arousal threshold and lowers the apnoea/hypopnoea index in obstructive sleep apnoea patients with a low arousal threshold. Clin Sci.

2011;120(12):505-514. https://doi.org/10.1042/CS20100588

[39] Smales ET, Edwards BA, Deyoung PN, McSharry DG, Wellman A, Velasquez A, Owens R, Orr JE, Malhotra A. Trazodone effects on obstructive sleep apnea and non-REM arousal threshold. Ann Am Thorac Soc. 2015;12(5):758-764. https://doi.org/10.1513/AnnalsATS.201408-399OC

[40] Chen, CY, Chen CL, Yu CC. Trazodone improves obstructive sleep apnea after ischemic stroke: a randomized, double-blind, placebo-controlled, crossover pilot study. J Neurol. 2021;268:2951-2960. https://doi.org/10.1007/s00415-021-10480-2

[41] Schifano F, Chiappini S, Corkery JM, Guirguis A. An insight into Z-drug abuse and dependence: an examination of reports to the European medicines agency database of suspected adverse drug reactions. International Journal of Neuropsychopharmacology. 2019;22(4):270-277. https://doi.org/10.1093/ijnp/pyz007

[42] Carter SG, Berger MS, Carberry JC, Bilston LE, Butler JE, Tong BKY, Martins RT, Fisher LP, McKenzie DK, Grunstein RR, Eckert DJ. Zopiclone increases the arousal threshold without impairing genioglossus activity in obstructive sleep apnea. Sleep. 2016;39(4):757-766. https://doi.org/10.5665/sleep.5622

[43] Wang D, Tang Y, Chen Y, Zhang S, Ma D, Luo Y, Li S, Su X, Wang X, Liu C, Zhang, N. The effect of non-benzodiazepine sedative hypnotics on CPAP adherence in patients with OSA: a systematic review and meta-analysis. Sleep. 2021;44(8), zsab077. https://doi.org/10.1093/sleep/zsab077

[44] Janto K, Prichard JR, Pusalavidyasagar S. An update on dual orexin receptor antagonists and their potential role in insomnia therapeutics. J Clin Sleep Med 2018;14(8):1399-1408. https://doi.org/10.5664/jcsm.7282

[45] Sakurai T. The neural circuit of orexin (hypocretin): maintaining sleep and wakefulness. Nat Rev Neurosci. 2007;8(3):171-181.

[46] Sun H, Palcza J, Card D, Gipson A, Rosenberg R, Kriger MLines C, Wagner JA, Troyer MD. Effects of suvorexant, an orexin receptor antagonist, on respiration during sleep in patients with obstructive sleep apnea. J Clin Sleep Med. 2016;12(1):9-17. https://doi.org/10.5664/jcsm.5382

[47] Eskandari D, Zou D, Grote L, Hoff E, Hedner J. Acetazolamide reduces blood pressure and sleep-disordered breathing in patients with hypertension and obstructive sleep apnea: a randomized controlled trial. J Clin Sleep Med. 2018;14(3):309-317. https://doi.org/10.5664/jcsm.6968

[48] Yang L, Zhang H, Cai M, Zou Y, Jiang X, Song L, Liang E, Bian J, Wu H, Hui R. Effect of spironolactone on patients with resistant hypertension and obstructive sleep apnea. Clinical and Experimental Hypertension. 2016;38:5, 464-468. https://doi.org/10.3109/10641963.2015.1131290

[49] Fiori CZ, Martinez D, Montanari CC, Lopez P, Camargo R, Sezera L, Goncavales SD, Fuchs FD. Diuretic or sodium-restricted diet for obstructive sleep apnea-a randomized trial. Sleep. 2018;41(4), zsy016. https://doi.org/10.1093/sleep/zsy016

[50] Furukawa S, Miyake T, Senba H, Sakai T, Furukawa E, Yamamoto S, Niiya T, Matsuura B, Hiasa Y. The effectiveness of dapagliflozin for sleep-disordered breathing among Japanese patients with obesity and type 2 diabetes mellitus. Endocr J. 2018;65(9):953-961. https://doi.org/10.1507/endocrj.EJ17-0545

[51] Tang Y, Sun Q, Bai XY, Zhou YF, Zhou QL, Zhang M. Effect of dapagliflozin on obstructive sleep apnea in patients with type 2 diabetes: a preliminary study. Nutr Diabetes. 2019;9(1):32. https://doi.org/10.1038/s41387-019-0098-5

[52] Taranto-Montemurro L, Messineo L, Sands SA, Azarbarzin A, Marques M, Edwards BA, Eckert DJ, White DP, Wellman A. The combination of atomoxetine and oxybutynin greatly reduces obstructive sleep apnea severity. A randomized, placebo-controlled, double-blind crossover trial. Am J Respir Crit Care Med. 2019;199(10): 1267-1276. https://doi.org/10.1164/rccm.201808-1493OC

[53] Horner RL, Grace KP, Wellman A. A resource of potential drug targets and strategic decision-making for obstructive sleep apnoea pharmacotherapy. Respirology. 2017;22(5):861-873. https://doi.org/10.1111/resp.13079

Section 4

Beyond the Pharmacotherapy of Sleep

Chapter 7

Sleep and the Fitness to Drive: A Swiss Perspective

Stefan Lakämper and Kristina Keller

Abstract

Medical conditions and behavioral patterns affecting sleep are a largely underestimated threat to traffic safety. Unsupervised or even illegal self-treatment of sleep issues by, for example, anti-histamines, cannabis products, or stimulants, questions safe driving and the fitness to drive as well as low compliance/adherence to treatments (CPAP, medication, etc.) of medical conditions, such as OSAS, or narcolepsy. In such cases, Swiss law calls for a medical assessment of the fitness to drive by experts in traffic medicine. With increasing complexity, this medical assessment is escalated in a four-tiered system of qualified experts, ranging from a qualified practitioner to experts in traffic medicine, at, for example, an Institute for Legal Medicine. The following overview provides insight in the Swiss framework of traffic medicine assessments that – with all caveats and potential drawbacks – helps mitigating the risk of sleep-related accidents. For this, we first introduce Swiss traffic medicine and then argue for consistent terms and measurements to assess sleepy driving. A concise summary of those sleep related conditions most relevant in traffic medicine is followed by an overview over potential issues of sleep-medication.

Keywords: sleep, fitness to drive, traffic medicine, OSAS, narcolepsy, sleep medication

1. Introduction

The consequences of medical conditions and behavioral patterns negatively affecting sleep pose a largely underestimated threat to traffic safety. According to a recent survey of Swiss road safety authorities (ASTRA), about 2% of all car accidents in Switzerland are documented to be caused unequivocally by the driver falling asleep [1]. Similar numbers are reported from other countries. The U.S. Institute for Insurance Information (III) lists "drowsy, asleep, fatigued, ill or blacked out" operation in 2.4% of drivers/operators involved in fatal crashes [2] and the U.S. National Highway Traffic Safety Administration (NHSTA) reports 1.9% of fatalities in motor vehicle crashes to have involved drowsy driving [3].

However, the estimated number of undetected or unreported accidents and fatalities might be much higher: various sources suspect that up to 30% of all accidents can be related – in part or full – to either falling asleep or to sleepiness at the wheel [4–6]. A study commissioned by the Australian Sleep Health foundation [7] and summarized prevalence and prevention information by the U.S. Center for Disease Control (CDC) [8] indicate that a surprisingly large fraction of the

IntechOpen

respective population suffers from undiagnosed sleep deprivation. In a representative poll, 1 in 25 U.S. adult drivers (ages 18 or older) report to have fallen asleep while driving in the last 30 days [9]. The NHSTA estimates that drowsy driving was responsible for 72,000 crashes, 44,000 injuries, and 800 deaths in 2013. These numbers are likely underestimated, and up to 6,000 fatal crashes each year may be caused by drowsy drivers in the U.S. alone [8, 10–12].

While the two preceding paragraphs illustrate the scope (of the threat/risk/challenge) with (impressive) figures, they also highlight a fundamental problem for mitigation strategies and concepts, i.e. an apparently incomplete definition and demarcation of terms used above, such as "drowsy, asleep, fatigued, ill, […] blacked out" [2], unconscious, tired, sleep-deprived or sleepy. The large spectrum of terms in use is in contrast to the need of a medical expert to communicated clearly and in a specific manner, not only with peers, but also in court, in assessments for authorities issuing driving licenses, and – last but not least – with his patients.

To briefly provide a few – possibly trivial, but illustrative – examples: it is essential if an unconscious patient caused an accident because he fell asleep or due a "black-out" (transient loss of consciousness, TLoC). Similarly, it is important whether a driver reports a "permanent subjective feeling of tiredness", or lacks any pre-sensation of spontaneously falling asleep in irregular intervals. While the latter might indicate narcolepsy, the first might possibly be very distracting from and dangerous for driving (inattention), but it might be short of any measurable danger to actually fall asleep. Chronic sleep-deprivation or sleep-fragmentation might lead to clearly measurable daytime sleepiness (excessive daytime sleepiness, EDS), but this might remain completely unnoticed to the driver. Over time, the driver's might have lost the ability to distinguish sleepiness from a (transient morning-) drowsiness or a post-prandial fatigue might have eroded, irrespective of the causes.

In the best case, any of the above conditions or situations is known ahead of any incident and family practitioners and experts in sleep- and traffic medicine collaborate for the best possible treatment and control to prevent any (daytime) sleepiness, in particular while driving.

However, one or more of the above situations or conditions might remain undetected, resulting, in the worst case, in an accident truly caused by the driver actually falling asleep. Such accidents, briefly termed sleep accident (SA) in the following text, usually exhibit certain characteristics. Drivers crash on a well-known monotonous road stretch, close to the final destination (e.g. home or work). Typically, there are no detectable traces of braking, of avoiding obstacles/vehicles or of abrupt changes in direction. In addition, drivers are usually well oriented and responsive in a clear and alert manner immediately following the accident [13]. However, indications are not always as clear and it is the second very mandate of traffic medicine to identify and document the causes of such accidents *post hoc*.

As already seen before, reasons for (daytime) sleepiness can be numerous and divers. Statistical figures hint at how one could structure a description of causes on a first level: the predominant fraction of SAs of drivers under 40 happen in weekend nights. In contrast, sleep accidents of drivers above 40 happen mostly on weekdays in the (late) afternoon [4]. Thus, following a dichotomization in "the younger partying" and "the older suffering from xx", the reasons can be divided very coarsely in predominantly behavioral or medical.

On a second level, the first might be further detailed in behavioral, social, professional and environmental reasons, whereas the latter might stem from central, neurological, somatic or psychiatric conditions or, finally, be substance- or medication-induced (See **Table 5**).

On a third level, that is also important for an overall assessment in traffic medicine, behavioral and social patterns overlaying fundamental causes might

Signs of sleep accident	**Signs of TLoC-accidents**
Monotonous, well known route	—
Close to destination	—
No trace of breaking	No trace of breaking
Immediately oriented driver	Continued disorientation
Diffuse knowledge about falling asleep	Despair about unclarity of causes
Rather trying to obscure clarifications	Strong interest in clarifying causes
Drivers aged <40: rather weekend nights	Independent of age
Drivers aged >40: rather afternoons	Independent of age
Seen by other drivers	**Seen by other drivers**
Slow reduction in speed	Abrupt changes in direction
Slowly loosing track	

Table 1.
Comparison of characteristic signs of sleep accidents as compared to accidents caused by a transient loss of consciousness (TLoC).

further aggravated the sleep conditions and associated risks in traffic. Especially in affluent and highly developed countries, with dense traffic and high social stress, sleep conditions are often counteracted by excessive use of commercially available stimulants (caffeine) or over the counter (OTC) substances (melatonin, doxylamine, diphenhydramine). Rather than addressing the problem, masking it by (an often inappropriate) use of such remedies already hampers mitigation of the risks. At the same time, several rounds of "next generation" sleep medication have repeatedly shown to involve the danger of developing tolerances, rebound- or side-effects, and even addiction. Especially latter is relevant in the context of self-medication and off label use of prescribed medication (antidepressants) or even drug abuse (cannabis, upper/downer, and opioids [14]), potentially causing unpredictable drug interactions leading to sudden sleepiness or TLoCs (**Table 1**).

The preceding paragraphs already outline the overall structure of the chapter and briefly sketch order and content of its sections: First, we introduce the unique set-up of Swiss traffic medicine, some necessary legal terms and recent organizational developments. We then argue for consistent use of terms and measurements used in the assessment of sleepiness. Following is a brief overview over those sleep conditions most relevant in every-day traffic medicine, including respective treatment options that are relevant to follow-up assessment. Lastly, we illustrate dangers of uninformed or inappropriate use of hypnotics and antidepressants due to drug interactions, highlighting the particular power of hair-analysis.

The chapter mostly collects regulations and existing literature. However, it is supplemented with two case reports and a short report on case numbers from the database of the division of traffic medicine at the Institute of Forensic Medicine at the University of Zurich.

2. Traffic medicine in Switzerland

To mitigate risks in traffic in general, Swiss license holders have to fulfill medical minimum requirements (MMR) by law (Strassenverkehrsgesetz, SVG Art 14 & 15 d, and Verkehrszulassungsverordnung, VZV, Art 7 [15, 16]). Swiss legislation already defined these "medical minimum requirements "(MMR) in 1932 in the form of ordinances [17]. These MMRs have been continuously modernized and adapted. In addition, they are framed by detailed subject-specific guidelines.

It is thus surprising that – despite known fatalities due to sleep accidents, the MMRs did, in fact, lack any explicit requirements with respect to sleep until 2016. Only then, a revision of the VZV in the context of a large-scale legislative effort to modernize and improve traffic (Via Sicura) specified in the MMR that there must not be any diseases or conditions leading to "elevated" daytime sleepiness. However, who does determine whether such a condition is or was present, and how? Are other contributing factors evaluated?

In general, the medical minimum requirements are controlled by experts trained in traffic medicine, who are organized and trained in a four-tiered federation-wide system, ranging from a trained physician (level 1) to full time experts (level 4, see **Figure 1**) since 2016.

Within this system, the medical assessment is escalated depending on the category of driving license applied for or increasing complexity, allowing for second opinions in doubt up to a level-4 expert, who are mostly associated with institutes for forensic/legal medicine. Among others, the law requires mandatory biannual checkups of elder drivers above age 75 for all categories and mandatory control exams for higher categories, such as professional taxi-, bus- or truck-drivers, after 3–5 years.

In the context of a sleep accident, the driver is in any case confronted with the question whether falling asleep – and thus the accident – happened in negligence; in other words, did the driver's behavior or wrongdoing lead to falling asleep or can it be attributed to a known or unknown medical condition. Apart from clarifying the legal issue of liability, this has direct consequences on the driver's license, as there are - at least – justified doubts whether the driver can fulfill the MMRs. In Swiss legal terms, it needs to be clarified whether the drivers momentary ability to drive (ATD, German: Fahrfähigkeit) or the drivers general fitness to drive (FTD, German: Fahreignung) was/or is given.

The legal term ability to drive (ATD,) refers to the driver's momentary and incidental physical and mental capabilities to safely conduct a vehicle. The ability to drive safely can be impaired by, for example, alcohol, improperly used medication and/or drugs. In addition, Swiss Federal Court rulings elaborate that in order for a driver to be legally "able to drive", both a basic capability and a mental and behavioral reserve capacity is required. This reflects the need to be able react adequately

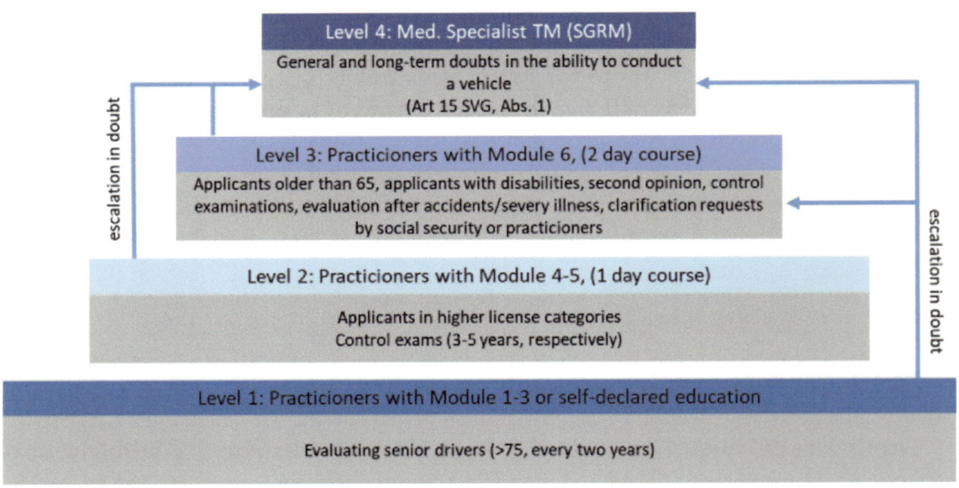

Figure 1.
Swiss four-tiered system of experts trained in traffic medicine.

to unexpected incidences in traffic and thus refers to the driver's requirement to guarantee this capacity before while driving, i.e. behavioral aspects, habits or character.

In contrast, the legal term "fitness to drive" (FTD) refers to the general physical and mental prerequisites to safely conduct a vehicle, unrelated to a specific incident or moment, relating obviously to chronic medical conditions limiting driving, which is in conflict with the MMRs. An assessment of the FTD or ATD at the level 3 or 4 generally encompasses a cursory medical examination (traffic medical exam, TME), anamnesis the patient's general medical status, history and recent incidents/events. Simple cognitive performance tests (mini mental status tests, clock test, trail making tests) reflect the need to take into account the general performance capabilities (German: Leistungsfähigkeit), assuming that safe driving requires both a basic physical and mental capacity (for undisturbed traffic, German: Grundleistung) as well as a mental and physical reserve capacity, relevant in unforeseen situations (German: Reserveleistung) [18].

While lower level assessments formally check general health, compliance, and adherence of, for example, the elderly drivers as required in two-year intervals at ages 75 and higher, higher-level assessments clearly deal with substantial doubts in the FTD, including those doubts relating to signs of addictive behavior and drug abuse. The final assessment provide the decision base for the authorities issuing the driving license.

According to recently updated guidelines [19], not all drivers who have caused a presumed sleep accident have to undergo a full TME and TMA in a top-tier institution (level 4): it is mandatory if there is information or hints pointing at either a medical condition or medication as the cause for falling asleep. In this case, the driving license is temporarily revoked until the authorities further decide based on the TMA. This is also the case, if it is unclear to both the driver and/or the authorities, whether the accident was truly caused by falling asleep or a transient loss of consciousness (TLoC, see Section 2.1) [20]. In case the driver can plausibly explain the accident by falling asleep due to behavior (too little sleep, shift work, etc.), a TMA is not required and subsequent sanctions by the authorities rely fully on the concession of an impaired driving ability.

2.1 Transient loss of consciousness as "camouflage statement" in sleep accidents

Because a first-time TLoC based on a so far unknown medical condition is presumed to have positive effects on the driver's liability assessment, a TLoC is often stated to "camouflage" any form misbehavior [21]. This is understandable in the context of patients that are, for example, very well aware of their own low medical or behavioral compliance/adherence, with known preconditions or psychogenic and gar-related cognitive deficits. Here, shame and the fear of consequences need to be taken into account.

A transient loss of consciousness (TLoC) as cause of an accident is already highly unlikely if during the anamnesis of the accident situation the above-mentioned characteristics can be found. However, this needs to be delimitated clearly; TLoCs can be caused by cerebral hypo-perfusion of cardiac, orthostatic or reflex origin, such as syncope, functional and medication arrhythmia, hypotonia, vasovagal reflexes hyper-responsive baroreceptor reflex in the carotid sinus or – without cerebral hypo-perfusion – by neurological, pharmacological or endocrinology conditions, such as epilepsy, narcolepsy, intoxication, hypoglycemia. In addition, a TLoC needs to be delimitated from other conditions such as a psychogenic pseudo-syncope, catatonia or cataplexy. The latter is often associated with narcolepsy and – in accident reconstruction – easily confused with falling asleep.

3. Sleepy driving: terms and measurements

The following section intends to take up the point of "incomplete definition and demarcation of terms used" as described in the introduction and tries to link a clarification to the legally binding - albeit slightly unclear - term "elevated daytime sleepiness" from the MMRs in Section 2, by arguing for ideally using consistent terms and measurements.

With "elevated daytime sleepiness" being the central term in Swiss legislation, this section, thus, clarifies our understanding of a.) Sleepiness (What are the signs of Sleepiness? What is sleepy? What is daytime sleepiness?) and b.) how to appropriately measure it? What is "elevated", "excessive" ... or – for that matter – "existing" (measurable) daytime sleepiness?

3.1 Sings of sleepiness

Fundamentally and independent of the time of day, measurement condition or cause, the state of "sleepy" displays unequivocal sings of imminent falling asleep. If the sleep needed is avoided - either willfully or by external force - these sings increase in frequency: if one is "sleepy", one yawns often and attack-like. Furthermore, it is increasingly difficult to keep the eyes open and these are often felt as "dry" and heavy ("heavy eyelids"). Muscle-tone and attention decrease significantly. Vision is reduced in focus and perception speed, often leading to blurred or even doubling pictures. In consequence, it becomes difficult to integrate environmental input correctly and to react to them in timely manner. At the same time, continued monotonous activities become erratic and concentrated. Sleepy test subjects also report on changed temperature sensation (rather towards chilly) and slightly increased perspiration (**Table 2**).

All these signs are believed to be noticed by all drivers [22, 23] well before influencing the driving performance significantly [24]. However, it remains unclear if, for example, chronically sleepy individuals (such as shift workers, truck drivers, etc.) are still able to correctly judge these signs and/or act accordingly. This might be influenced by continued willful ignorance and, thus, familiarization/desensibilisation.

As mentioned above, there exists a general uncertainty as to how discriminate the state of "sleepiness" from terms that are used in a similar or even synonymous way: these include tiredness, exhaustion and drowsiness (see below). Lastly, the difficulty to actually "measure" and "communicate a measure" of sleepiness should not be underestimated, even in the medical and diagnostic context. Therefore, the following section aims at clarifying terms and measures used in Swiss traffic medicine.

3.2 Measures of sleepiness and its relevance in traffic medicine

As clarified in the preceding section, sleepiness *per se* is a natural reaction: it is the direct presage of the functional and unavoidable necessity to sleep, as dictated by chronobiology in (more or less) regular intervals, normally in the evening [23, 25, 26]. Therefore and irrespective of the cause, be it medical or behavioral, the customary composite "day-time sleepiness" describes an unusual and, in traffic, inacceptable condition.

Signs of sleepiness
Yawning (repeated, in attacks)
Dry eyes
«heavy eye lids
Sharp vision requires effort
Reduced muscle tone
Reduced attention, effort for vigilance strongly increased
Changed temperature sensation
Sweating (forehead)
Consequences for perception and performance in general
Visual perception slowed down and blurred
Slowed and error prone integration of environmental influences
Monotonous actions/tasks increasingly erratic and unconcentrated
Effects on driving performance
Track and speed cannot be held constant
Unexpected reduction of speed, inexplicable for others
Abrupt corrections of speed and direction when waking up

Table 2.
Unequivocal signs of being sleepy at the wheel.

Independent of the time of day, "sleepiness" also describes an initially abstract measure of the inclination or tendency to fall asleep [27]. Transferred in a concrete and manageable measurement, this measure is operationally defined as the recorded time from a test start until a test subject actually falls asleep (in minutes), i.e. a latency. This parameter is also termed "sleep latency", but requires the actual test situation to be named (see below). Although seemingly intuitive, but slightly incorrectly, this parameter is also circumscribed as "sleep propensity" (**Figure 2**).

Figure 2(a) displays a schematic course of performance change during the day in % (after [23]). Based on this, **Figure 2(b)** illustrates the measurement of sleep latencies and allows clarifying the difference between the terms sleep latency and sleep propensity (sleep inclination). Solid lines in red or blue, respectively, illustrate schematically the "course" (on an arbitrary, qualitative scale ranging from "awake" to "asleep") from the start of the test (t = 0) until the test subject has fallen asleep (crossing the x-axis). L1-L3 indicate three different sleep latencies. It is apparent that on red and blue solid lines each result in the same sleep latency, but starting from a different (abstract and qualitative) activity level. The dashed red and blue lines, four of which are denoted as N1-N4, indicate the slopes (inclinations) resulting from start and end of the measurements. N1-N4 help to illustrate the slightly misleading term sleep propensity/inclination: given the same latency L1, N1 shows a steep slope, N2 displays a flat slope, as it starts form a lower activity level. N2 is similar to N3, which relates to a much longer latency L3. Vice versa, N4 is much smaller as compared to N3 although it corresponds to the same Latency L3. As the latency has been made accessible through operationalization, the activity level remains fully elusive. Consequently, the terms sleep inclination/propensity should be avoided in favor of the clearly defined sleep latency. The same applies to terms such as sleep pressure for which an illustrative correlate is even harder to find.

Sleep latencies are usually measured in two ways, the MSLT and the MWT [28]. Most frequent in sleep medicine is the classical multiple sleep latency test (MSLT).

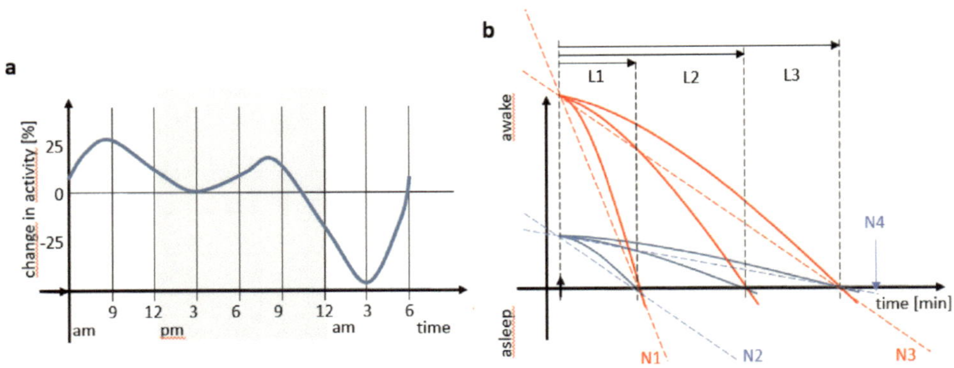

Figure 2.
(a) Schematic course of performance change during the day in % (after [23]). (b) Three exemplary courses of activity from awake to asleep form two different starting levels (red and blue) including measured sleep latencies (L1–L3, black arrows)). N1–4 (red and blue dashed lines) illustrate slopes (inclinations) to argue against the terms sleep inclination or sleep propensity (see main text).

In four or five repetitions at intervals of 2 h, it is observed, if - and how fast - a test subject is falling asleep within 20 min. Individuals are subjected to a typical sleep setting: she/he is lying in a bed in a fully darkened room with closed eyes and with the purpose to fall asleep. Once the EEG registers a > 15 s stretch of one or more of the three typical sleep states, the measurement stops and the individual is woken up. Final MSLT sleep latency is the average of the 4–5 measurements. The MSLT thus measures how fast a test subject can manage to fall asleep during the day.

The multiple wakefulness test (MWT) measures also a sleep latency, but approaches sleepiness from the opposite perspective, i.e. the wish to stay awake. Individuals are subjected to a soporific, but not ideal situation: she/he is sitting in a comfortable chair in a partially darkened (dim) room with open eyes and with the clear purpose not to fall asleep, i.e. to stay awake. Again, the above-mentioned 15 s-rule for the EEG applies to determine after how long an individual has fallen asleep within either 20 min. or - more usual - 40 min. Again, this latency is measured in four or five repetitions with intervals of 2 h. Final MWT sleep latency is the average of the 4–5 measurements. The MWT thus measures, how many minutes a person can (actively) avoid falling asleep during the day. The MWT includes active elements and incorporates the ability of the test subject to counteract falling asleep. Consequently, the MWT is considered more comparable to assessing a driving situation than the MSLT [28, 29].

However, clinicians might use definitions of EDS and criteria of it in MWT/ MSLT differing from or overlapping with those in traffic medicine [28]. The new ICSD-3 [30, 31] defines EDS as "daily episodes of an irrepressible need to sleep or daytime lapses into sleep". For disorders, such as narcolepsy and idiopathic hypersomnia (IH), which require demonstration of objective sleepiness by the multiple sleep latency test (MSLT), a mean sleep latency of 8 min on the MSLT is required. This criterion is unchanged from the ICSD-2 and represents the best compromise between sensitivity and specificity [32]. Here, the MWT is not specifically mentioned as diagnostic tool, while its relevance in the clinic has been proven useful for the evaluation of treatment success with respect to everyday life situations [28].

Swiss guidelines for traffic medical assessments allow for a modification of the MWT, in slight favor of the drivers, the FTD-MWT: here is allowed to consume usual amounts of beverages containing caffeine during breaks and to take one mid-day nap of 20 min. Both is not allowed in the diagnostic classical MSLT and MWT. In practice, the number of modified FDT-MWTs is, however, very low.

In order to discriminated daytime sleepiness as measured predominantly by MWTs from an increased demand of sleep due to neurological conditions, such as a hypersomnia or a narcolepsy [28], the MWT is usually accompanied by polysomnography (PSG, classic, ad libitum) which should ideally follow directly after a 14-day period of actigraphy, including protocolling the sleep behavior [29].

Such "objective" measures of sleepiness as measured in MWT or MSLT should be clearly distinguished from phenomenological experienced and questionnaire-based, i.e. "subjective" sleepiness. Some questionnaires and methods (KSS, as well as VAS-batteries), determined a "momentary and felt" sleepiness, whereas, for example, the ESS determines the subjective estimate of sleepiness over a period of time (usually 14 days) post hoc and in relation to representative situations and, therefore, registers - at best - an average subjective feeling. Although often in use, the ESS is strongly criticized for is high level of subjectivity [27]. Also, the ESS offers low prognostic reliability, as the subjective estimate of sleepiness might manifest differently in different, soporific situations, such as monotonous night drives or similar [33].

3.3 Day-time sleepiness: qualifiers and guidelines

It is the very nature of the so-far mentioned tests that, in principle, they can measure both the natural sleepiness induced by medical conditions and behavioral patterns, both in the course of the day and at night. *In realiter*, these tests are almost exclusively performed and related to the common daytime period, in order to evaluate deviation from the norm.

Intermittent or chronic sleepiness during the day as measured by way of above-mentioned objective methods is termed "daytime sleepiness". However, in different contexts the term is often complemented with varying qualifying adjectives: to state two, the medical field generally prefers the term "excessive daytime sleepiness" (EDS) [34] mostly in connection with insomnias and other conditions. As introduced in Section 2, Swiss law prohibits driving with medical conditions leading to any "elevated" (German: erhöhte) daytime sleepiness. Other qualifiers "significantly increased", "relevant", "excessive" and "severe" daytime sleepiness, leaving the reader often without respective information how to understand and value the qualifier. German regulations have taken up this issue by clarifying that "any measurable" daytime sleepiness is relevant to the assessment of the fitness to drive. In this meaning, but for reasons of general understanding, we here continue using the general term EDS.

Contrary to sleepiness (both in general and EDS), the concepts of "tiredness", "exhaustion" or even "fatigue", often originating from a very broad spectrum of psychogenic and chronic syndromes, are not very well accessible to latency measurements. Apparently, latency measures – especially MSLT-measurements – produce even paradox information: while physical activity improves (i.e. reduces) daytime sleepiness, the very broad and rather unspecific "tiredness" in the above mentioned syndromes is aggravated by physical activity, but cannot me measured in MSLT and MWT as these monotonous and soporific test situations do not represent a stimulus for sleep [35].

In consequence, the assessment of the fitness to drive in the case of a chronic medical condition relating to sleep critically hinges on evaluating daytime sleepiness (EDS) by way of MWT sleep-latency measurements. This is particularly important in order to assess treatment progress and/or treatment compliance.

Current guidelines provide orientation to assess the fitness to drive as based on MWT sleep latencies (**Table 3**). *Per definitionem* the MWT captures daytime sleepiness (EDS) at values <40 min. Empirical and normative data display that 97.5% of

Fitness to drive (lower categories)	**Positive**	**Borderline positive**	**Borderline negative**	**Negative**
MWT latency (average)	≥ 34 min	20–33 min		< 20 min
MWT latency (single)				< 20 min
single sleep fragments (<5 s)	normal	normal		
Multiple sleep fragments (<5 s)			X (repetition)	
Longer sleep fragments (>5 s)			X (repetition)	
Fitness to drive (higher categories)	**Positive**	**Borderline positive**	**Borderline negative**	**Negative**
MWT latency (average)	≥ 34 min			< 34 min
Any sleep fragements				X (6 month)

Table 3.
Evaluation of the fitness to drive based on MWT-sleep latencies and other parameters as measure in an MWT according to current guidelines [10].

healthy test subjects can stay awake for more than 8 min and 59% for 40 min or more [33, 36]. Current guidelines suggest a limiting MWT sleep latency of ≥34 min as the limit to a relevant "excessive daytime sleepiness" (EDS), corresponding well with the average sleep latency of 36.5 min [28]. However, the guidelines allow leeway in as far as single sleep fragments and micro-sleep episodes might be allowed, although their existence strongly recommends repeating the MWT after a reduced control interval and/or improved therapy.

4. Relevant conditions in traffic medicine

As has become clear in Section 2 of this chapter, traffic medicine is – in some way - a statutory service institution. Assessments are by order of (and paid for by) the driver but serve the issuing authorities in deciding if or under which conditions a driving license can be (re)-granted. The assessment covers all medical fields (see MMR). While unclear conditions or problems might prompt further inquiries to associated specialists, Traffic medicine is far from being a diagnostic or a treatment institution, but rather a "medical detective's office".

This position encompasses, that a broad knowledge, long-term experience and a keen eye/ear for potential inconsistencies in the stories told by drivers form the basis of – often very standard and uniform - daily assessments and control exams.

This includes also, that many of the more severe or chronic conditions are, in fact, managed by the family physician and associated specialists. Higher-level expert in traffic medicine might thus check and confirm a lower level assessment of a managing doctor based on records and statements, but might not see the patient directly. To give an example unrelated to this books topic, a well-controlled diabetic is only rarely required to undergo a level 4 exam. Similarly, well-documented state of treatment positive and compliant patients with affective disorders are sufficient.

The same applies to the large field of conditions affecting sleep: Severe conditions immediately prompt the action of specialists and might lead to immediate revocation of a driver's license, be it permanent or until successful treatment is documented according to guidelines. With respect to sleep conditions, it is rather the unclear cases, *post hoc* assessments of accidents and substance/medication-related issues – mostly involving the danger of EDS – that are present in traffic medicine.

4.1 Conditions leading to EDS

It is evident from the preceding chapters, that the symptom of a measurable daytime-sleepiness (EDS) stemming from either behavioral aspects or medical conditions is most relevant to traffic medicine in the assessment of the fitness to drive. In the following section, we provide a brief overview over the prevalence and the different medical conditions associated with EDS.

For lack of a general public health definition of EDS accessible to large-scale public health studies, the determination of the prevalence of EDS has proven to be difficult. With estimated prevalence ranging between 3.2 to 32.5% as reported in [37], valuable information for orientation is provided by yearly polls of the U.S. National Sleep Foundation [38]. The 2008 poll reports, that around 30% of participants concede to sleepy/drowsy driving at least once per month during the last year, mostly to and from work ([39], p. 32). While this number is highly subjective, ESS-data provide a slightly less subjective or more systematic orientation about self-assessed sleepiness: accordingly, 18% of the participants scored 10 or more points qualifying them as excessively sleepy with increased likelihood of medical conditions [40]. A more stringent report [37] analyzed data from 5,962 face-to face interviews within the National Comorbidity Survey Replication (NCS-R), resulting in a prevalence of EDS of 23%. This study identified individuals with significant impairment/distress due to "excessive sleepiness (ExS.)" based on reported sleepiness in conjunction with an irrepressible need for sleep, difficulty waking up and/or prolonged nighttime sleep that was unrefreshing [37].

In **Table 4**, we summarized and categorized possible origins for EDS by (a) Sleep deprivation, i.e. too little sleep in general, be it behavioral or situational, (b) Reasons for fragmented sleep be it for environmental or medical reasons, (c) Primary CNS related hypersomnia, including narcolepsy, (d) "True" neurological conditions that might be associated directly or indirectly with altered sleep e.) Psychiatric conditions often accompanied directly or indirectly with altered sleep and, lastly, (recreational or illicit) substances/stimulants or medications that typically induce EDS and/or sleepiness. Due to its focus on the outcome sleepiness, rather the table might seem somewhat arbitrary. However, this categorization should not be confused with a classification of sleeping disorders *per se* as in, for example [42], or the new ICSD-3 [30–32].

We therefore added coloring, indicating items in different categories that are accessible to similar treatment/changes. Accordingly, basically all reasons for sleep deprivation, sleep fragmentation by environmental reasons and most substance induced reasons for sleepiness/EDS are accessible to behavioral/situational change (light blue) Obstructive sleep apnea syndrome and Obesity Hypoventilation Syndrome are accessible to device assisted treatment (CPAP, APAP, servo ventilation, gray).

While narcolepsy and epilepsy are often well manageable with relatively mild medication (light red), many primary CNS hypersomnia and neurological conditions, including RLS and PLMD are less accessible to treatment or require more complex care management (gray-blue). Similarly, the most other organic conditions require complex medication including symptomatic pain relief (yellow, see opiates). Lastly, care and medication psychiatric conditions requires specialized attention with respect to EDS and sleepiness, in particular in the context of the fitness to drive (light green).

(a) Sleep deprivation	(b) Fragmentation of sleep	(c) Primary CNS hypersominas	(d) Neurological conditions	(e) Other organic causes	(f) Psychiatric conditions	(g) Substance or medication induced
Behavioral pattern	Obstructive sleep apnea syndrome	Narcolepsy	Neurodegenerative disorders (Parkinson Alzheimer)	Congestive heart failure	Depression and other affective disorders	Alcohol
Sleep hygiene	Restless leg syndrome	Idiopathic hypersomnia	Multiple Sclerosis	Chronic renal failure	Anxiety disorders	Stimulant overdose/ withdrawal (Nicotine, caffeine)
Altered sleep phases	Periodic limb movement disorder	Parasomnias	Stroke	Liver failure	Psychotic disorders	Sleeping pills
Jet lag	Environmental disturbances (noise, light)	Cyclic or episodic hypersomnia	Epilepsy	Malineoplastic and malignancy syndromes	Post-traumatic stress disorders	Drug abuse (Cannabis, cocaine)
Shift work	Central sleep apnea syndrome	Menstrual-related sleep disorder	CNS tumors	Obesity hypoventilation syndrome		Opiates, Benzodiazepines, Barbiturates
Stress, voluntary sleep rejection		Kleine-Levin Syndrome				Anti-epileptics, Gamma-Hydroxy-Butyrate (Xyrem)
						Antidepressant, Neuroleptic

Table 4.
Common causes of and contributors to EDS/sleepiness (modified after [41]).

As the occurrence of EDS is trivial or at least likely in cases of hypersomnia or neurological disorders, respectively, specialist case management addresses this danger usually in a very efficient manner. Consequently, traffic medicine rarely receives unclear cases stemming from these conditions. Rather, traffic medicine is usually only required to assess and document the requirement for regular reports of lower level experts - in most cases the patient's physician - to the authorities.

EDS can be caused, on the one hand, by short- or long-term (miss-) behavior (i.e. "partying) or working conditions such as night or shift work [43]. On the other hand, it can stem from medical conditions, such as narcolepsy [44], hypersomnia [45], OSAS [46], RLS [47], or medication, such as anti-histaminica or antidepressants [48, 49]. In the clinical setting, two of the most commonly encountered causes leading to EDS are obstructive sleep apnea, restless leg syndrome and periodic limb movement disorder [41]. Other reports count non-apnea sleep disorders higher in risk, but for all injuries, not limited to driving [50]. At the same time, several reports [51] indicate, that also sleep medication- or sleep medication-withdrawal-induced psychomotor impairments/disorders, such as REM-sleep behavior disorder, RBD, might lead to parasomnias and, in consequence, EDS [42].

While our own records indicate only 114 out of 256,387 entries indicate a clear sleep accident (search term "Einschlafunfall") of various origins, we do find 750 and 1,904 entries for the term OSAS or sleep apnea (search term "Schlafapnoe"), respectively 170 entries are retrieved for sleeping problems (search term "Schlafstörung"), 125 for restless-leg syndrome and 111 entries for narcolepsy. Only 17 entries can be retrieved for hypersomnia.

The potentially multifactorial origin of EDS shows exemplarily the importance of a full anamnesis and complete medical examination in traffic medicine. We illustrate this by way of a case study.

4.2 Case study 1: uncovering a case of OSAS-induced EDS

One morning in March, around 7 am, a 62-year-old man drove at moderate speed on a straight street to work. According to eyewitnesses, the driver's car moved more and more towards the lane of the oncoming traffic. After two small grazing collisions, a frontal collision at moderate speed ended the drive. The driver reported a "blackout" and declared no recollection of the initial grazing collisions or ignition of the airbags. He reported to be "fully back" immediately after the frontal crash. He stepped out of the car unharmed, called the police helped the other driver and secured the site. Subsequently, a "wave-like" uneasiness with low pulse (40 bps) set in, which lasted for around 3 hours. As neither he nor the police could clearly identify a sleeping incident and he claimed a blackout, the police revoked his driving license based on a first-time TLoC until final assessment in traffic medicine. He was hospitalized for 3 days for both security and further check-ups.

For the traffic medical exam, which took place 5 months later in August, the patient presented himself in good physical and mental conditions. He reported to be in good health, to have been active, to drink usual amounts of alcohol and to be fully drug-naïve. He reported plans to retire abroad the following year after 40 years of successful work. He is unable to explain the blackout, as he has driven this route to work about "100,000 times".

Extensive medical exams included cardiological, neurological and neuro-angiological reports, including overnight EEG. While epileptiform spike-patters were observed when falling asleep, these were considered norm variants and not to causative for a blackout. However, strong snoring and a medium-grade OSAS was reported with an AHI of 33 although this was restricted to unusual sleeping positions (back). The patient was surprised about this finding and reported to notice no negative physical effects of this condition. Only, his wife moved out of the bedroom due to the snoring. As there was no evidence excluding a TLoC and indication for an OSAS – although without clear signs of EDS – the permission to drive was not re-granted. This assessment could be reconsidered, provided the patient had proof for no further TLoC-like events within a year and could provide a repeated polysomnographic examination for confirmation of the moderate state of his OSAS.

The patient presented himself 13 months later (September) with the following records: A second PSG (performed December the previous year) reported a severe OSAS with AHI of 77, ESS 3/27 with subjectively normal sleep. At this point, a MWT was performed, but was considered non-evidentiary, such that there is no result reported. APAP treatment was initiated in January. An MWT performed in May confirmed inconspicuous (4 x > 40 min) with very good patient compliance. The snoring had subsided and the wife had moved back into the shared bedroom. Despite clear signs for a sleep accident, the initial round of examinations only revealed unclear results, except indications for an un-diagnosed sleep condition (OSAS) from the wife's reports and a first nighttime-EEG. Here the patient's compliance is exemplary. Based on this and no further indication of a TLoC-like event, the assessment supported re-granting the license on the condition of yearly follow-up reports. Most likely due to his retirement and relocation abroad the patient was lost to follow-up in our files.

In conclusion, it is in the interest of the individual driver's safety and traffic safety in general to obtain a full anamnesis and medical examination in traffic medicine. While traffic medicine is primarily neither a diagnostic nor therapeutic instance, traffic medicine's unique perspective, mandate and its concomitant in-depth assessment of the medical fitness to drive allows detecting previously unreported cases of EDS.

However, an EDS based on medical condition might be obscured or – vice versa - incorrectly assumed, when other conditions require medication that potentially leads to sleepiness. This will be highlighted in the following chapter that introduces the dimension of depression, age and behavior in the context of inappropriate use of medication, such as antidepressants and sleeping pills.

5. Substance (ab/mis)use and the fitness to drive

As outlined in Section 2, active participation in traffic requires adequate physical and psychological performance and reserve capacities. With any medication or substance taken, one's overall performance might improve or worsen. While many substances might reduce performance in a noticeable, but manageable fashion, some might induce (daytime) sleepiness. This is particularly true for most psychoactive substances, either in its wanted or unwanted effects (such as lag, hangover, rebound, side effects, and paradox reactions).

Somewhat trivial but not always known, this is clearly true for sleeping pills, (hypnotics/ hypnosedativa), but also for medication in psychiatric disorders (antidepressants, antipsychotics), allergies (antihistaminic) and, partially, degenerative disorders (e.g. Parkinson) [52]. Therefore, traffic medicine needs to know how to evaluate the fitness and the ability to drive under the influence of such medication. As described in the first paragraphs of this section, this is particularly important if such medication is combined, as often – but not exclusively - the case of elderly drivers.

We then provide a brief sketch of historic improvements and persisting problems of the above classes of drugs, with a focus on potential issues for safe driving related to sleep, leading general recommendations for experts based on a classification by the International Council on Alcohol, Drugs and Traffic Safety, ICADTS. Subsequently we evaluate potential issues of excessive self-medication (melatonin, doxylamine) and the (ab)use of (illicit) drugs such as cannabis, barbiturates and opioids. By way of a case example, we highlight the value of hair sampling for controlling long-term substance (ab)use.

5.1 The triangle depression, sleep, and age

According to a recent report of the Swiss health observatory (Obsan) from 2016 [53], a substantial fraction of the Swiss population feels heavily (5%) or moderately to heavily (13%) burdened with mental and psychological problems. Consequently, 18 out of 100 are likely to present mental disorders. Yearly prevalence varies by year: most frequent are anxiety disorders (14%), affective disorders (7.8%), somatoform disorders (4.9%) and alcohol-related disorders (3.4%). Almost 90% of all affective disorders are depressions (6.9% of total). Around 5% of the Swiss population take either hypnotics on a daily basis. About 40% of the population with mental problems take antidepressants. In both groups, women are more prevalent, and the incidence increases strongly with age [54]. Importantly, there are indications that there is a gender difference in driving performance when using hypnotic medication [55].

While antidepressants alone might have strong effects on driving performance via sleep disturbance [14], initial symptom of above mentioned mental disorders (or of the prolonged stress periods leading to mental disorders), is heavily disturbed sleep, directly linking an increased use and prescription of psychopharmaca to that of hypnotic medication, i.e. sleeping pills, the latter often being benzodiazepines or Z-Drugs [53].

These figures have increased in the last decades [56] and steep increases in these figures are to be expected as a consequence of the severe social restriction due to the corona pandemic. Here, sleep patterns that are altered due to the lack of social control (school, home-office, retirement and lack of social contacts) might themselves contribute to the etiology of psychiatric disorders and stress-syndromes, in particular in children and adolescents. Conversely, the demographic increase of elderly drivers with increasing rates of comorbidities and concomitant multi-medication might potentiate the relevance of drug interactions in traffic on the other side of the age spectrum. However, even without age-related conditions or depression, the elderly often report sleep issues, which are loosely remedied by standard hypnotics, such as Z-Drugs and benzodiazepines, or self-medication by off label use [57].

Here, many patients naively presume that prescribed or OTC medication does not pose a risk in traffic and do not even mention taking it in an assessment. Similarly, the addictive potential of some of the medication and "doctor hopping" to obtain a desired drug should not be underestimated, even in highly regulated markets such as Switzerland. Such unmonitored self-medication might result in adverse side effects and unexpected drug interactions.

5.2 General recommendation for prescribing doctors and classification of medication

In any case, the above unknowns poses a series of problems for both prescribing doctors and experts in traffic medicine. Whenever assessing the FTD or prescribing new medication experts should answer the following set of questions:

- Does a medication have positive and/or negative effects on physical and mental performance and reserve capacity required for safe driving, and if yes, how much? Is the result balanced?

  In other words: Does the medications main effect sufficiently increase physical and mental performance and reserve capacity required for safe driving? Do the medication's undesired effects lower the physical and mental performance and reserve capacity required for safe driving?

- How long the medication should be prescribed?

- Are there long-term consequences of the treatment (Parkinson, L-Dopa, wear-off effects), indicating negative progression and thus narrower control intervals of the FTD?

- Is there addictive potential associated with the drug?

- Is the medication taken correctly? Are compliance and adherence given?

- Do any indications exist, that call for checking adherence/compliance by blood-level testing or similar?

While information relating medication to accident risks or odds ratios exists [57], it is limited and painstaking to collect. However, both on the acute level (i.e. the ability to drive) and the long term (the fitness to drive) it is widely undisputed that psychotropic drugs do affect the capabilities for safe driving: very simply speaking, hypnotic, sedatives and antidepressants are prescribed to calm down, to lower activity level and/or to fall asleep. It seems, on the one hand, thus, rather trivial that these desired effects might have spill-over-effects of the ability to drive.

It is not trivial on the other hand, to collect and categorize the existence and, subsequently, the extent of such effects on safe driving. Thankfully, the large-scale EU-Project DRUID (Driving Under the Influence of Drugs) that included participation of the ICADTS presented an aggregated list of medications affecting safe driving [58, 59] and published according prescription guidelines [57].

Listed drugs were classified as follows:

I. Presumed to be safe or unlikely to produce an effect

II. Likely to produce minor or moderate adverse effects

III. Likely to produce severe effects or presumed to be potentially dangerous

All antidepressants/-psychotics and hypnotics are listed in category II or III. The most relevant drugs are listed in **Table 5**, possibly a helpful tool for both physicians and experts.

Wherever know, detailed information is provided as to how long not to drive after changes in the respective medication. As a general rule of thumb from the perspective of traffic medicine, patients should abstain from driving for a period of about 14 days after treatment start, change or end of a treatment regime.

With every change in medication, the effects of prescribed drugs as well as the duration of effects on driving should be explained in detail. The recommendation to abstain from driving and the warning information should be registered in the

Active ingredient	Classification	Active ingredient	Classification
ANTIPSYCHOTICS		**BENZODIAZEPINES + Z-DRUGS**	
Levomepromazine	III	Diazepam	III
Fluphenazine	II	Chlordiazepoxide	III
Perphenazine	II	Oxazepam	III
Thioridazine	III	Potassium clorazepate	II
Haloperidol	II	Lorazepam	III
Melperone	II	Bromazepam	III
Pipamperone	II	Alprazolam	III
Benperidol	II	Flurazepam	III
Flupentixol	II	Nitrazepam	III
Zuclopentixol	II	Flunitrazepam	III
Clozapine	II	Triazolam	III
Olanzapine	II	Lormetazepam	III 1 mg (capsule): >10 hours post dosing little or no impairment (Category I)
Quetiapine	II	Temazepam	III 10 mg: >10 hours post dosing little or no impairment (Category I)
Sulpiride	II	Midazolam	III
Amisulpride	II	Zopiclon	III
Lithium	II	Zolpidem	II 10 mg: >10 hours post dosing little or no impairment (Category I)
Risperidone	II	Zaleplon	II 10 mg: >5 hours post dosing little or no impairment (Category I)
Clotiapine	II		
ANTI-DEPRESSANTS		**ANTI-DEPRESSANTS**	
Desipramine	II	Paroxetine	I
Imipramine	II	Sertraline	I
Clomipramine	II	Fluvoxamine	I
Trimipramine	III	Escitalopram	I
Amitriptyline	III	Moclobemide	I
Nortriptyline	II	Mianserin	III
Doxepin I	II	Trazodone	III
Melitracen	II	Mirtazapine	III
Fluoxetine	I	Venlafaxine	I
Citalopram	I		
		STIMULANTS	
		Dexamfetamine	II
		Methylphenidate	II

Table 5.
Classification of hypnotics, anti-depressants and -psychotics, stimulants with respect to effects on driving according to the DRUID study [58] in collaboration with ICADTS [60]. Excerpt from [59].

patient's records. After the initial treatment phase, patients should be controlled. If there are clinical sings of, for example generally lowered response time, reduced vigilance, reduced speed of perception processing or motoric effects, the patient should not be allowed to drive as these severely affect the reserve capacity for safe driving substantially.

In particular, drugs carrying an addictive potential should not be prescribed for long terms and their appropriate (therapeutic) dosage and use should be confirmed by blood-level testing.

5.3 Disappointed and false expectations: sleep medication and its effect on driving in a historical perspective

Disturbances of sleep have always troubled humanity [61]. Sleep medicine as a subject field in medicine has only evolved rather late (c. since the mid 1970s) but fulminant [62]. This especially after linking mayor breakthroughs in measurement technologies, findings and concepts such as the electroencephalogram, EEG [63], detection of sleep-stages [64] including rapid eye movement sleep, REM, [65], to the regulation and control of circadian rhythms and chronobiology [26, 66, 67].

Before bromides solutions emerged in the 1800s, it was mostly alcohol and drugs such as opium and cannabis that served to induce or facilitate falling asleep. The first effective synthetic hypnotic was chloral hydrate in 1869, followed by paraldehyde around 1880 and the introduction of the first of a long series of barbiturates (phenobarbital, 1912) after initial synthesis of the founding compound barbital in 1903.

While the above substances were introduced well before the public had widespread access to such medication or, for that matter, driving, their addictive potential and recreational use remain a problem in traffic medicine today.

Between the first and second world war, the extensive, indiscriminate and uncontrolled use of barbiturates (and for that matter other drugs [68]) such as, phenobarbital, secobarbital, amobarbital and pentobarbital in the general population coincides with an increase of cars and traffic density.

This increase in cars and traffic density accelerated drastically with the beginning of the second half of the 20th century, motivating a further evolution of traffic medicine, more and more including the control of addictive substances. This development parallels a boost in the development in sleep medicine (see above) but also coincides with the development and increasingly widespread use of the next generation of hypnotics, the benzodiazepines, which today are still one of the most widely prescribed group of medication.

The lower number of unfavorable side effects of benzodiazepines as compared to barbiturates led to brad use as a household hypnotic, severely underestimating the development of tolerances, addiction and side effects. As above mentioned for early sleep remedies, the (by-)use of benzodiazepines in recreational settings keeps this class of hypnotic well in the focus of traffic medicine even nowadays [14].

Much like in other, earlier cases (radium, heroin, pervitin [68]) the repeated promise of "side-effect-free" medicine proved to be naïve and incorrect again. In particular, benzodiazepines are associated with a rather large number of psychomotor disorders indirectly affecting sleep in a negative way [51].

Initially, this seemed to be different with a new group of hypnotics, arriving in the late 1980ies: the non-benzodiazepines, often called Z-Drugs [69], promised to be specific and highly effective hypnotics. However, identical pharmacodynamics as compared to benzodiazepines indicate paths to similar side effects. These are, however, sometimes slightly less pronounced or just different: Z-Drugs seem to have lower tendency for physical dependence and addiction, but are known to produce amnesia and, rarely, hallucinations. Counterintuitively, some of the Z-Drugs double the risk of developing depression and some long-terms studies found a marked increase in suicide risk [70]. Zolpidem itself is associated with rebound insomnia, possibly resulting in subsequently aggravated EDS. In Contrast to zolpidem and zopiclone, zalepon is not associated with an increased risk of motor vehicle accidents [71]. However, effects of Z-Drugs on human performance including some rather bizarre behavioral effects heavily affecting sleep have been summarized [69].

Nowadays, swift and thorough testing the effects of novel - and supposedly again more specific - hypnotics on driving performance [72] prevents major surprises in novel sleep medication with respect to effects on driving performance. This includes orexin system blockers, such as Suvorexant [73] and Lemborexant [74], or melatonin agonists [66, 67], such as Ramelteon [71, 75].

This also applies to reevaluation of older information [76, 77] concerning driving performance after the "rediscovery" of some tricyclical antidepressants, such as doxepin (Silenor) [78] which effectively trigger sleep onset in an antihistamine-like fashion, i.e. by selectively blocking H1-receptors.

As mentioned above for the older generations of dedicated hypnotics, older generations of other medication have been - and are still - used to facilitate or induce sleep based on their side effects. However, the negative consequences on driving performance might however be even more pronounced than in modern hypnotics. Depending on a countries medical system, this self-medication is more or less uncontrolled. Here in particular, ab- or miss-use of over the counter drugs might be risky in traffic. Additionally, some of these substances are likely to be part of an addictive behavior. Some substances have even become literally "traditional" to the degree of "folklore". To mention here directly are, among others, first-generation antihistamines such as doxylamine (e.g. Sanalepsi, Unisom), diphenhydramine (e.g. Benadryl, Nytol), but also partially available antitussives such as codeine (e.g. Mucatussin) but also the inappropriate use of melatonin pills with questionable results on sleep, but potentially sever impacts on driving performance [79–81].

With this plethora of information to deal with, it is to be expected that unintended and uniformed misuse of individual or combined medication might lead to sleepiness on the wheel, potentially resulting in severe accidents. Similar to unknown medical conditions, it is again traffic medicine's mandate to "elucidate" the exact or at least most likely cause of such accidents. Very often a thorough anamnesis and sighting of all available records is insufficient to give conclusive results. It is then, that modern tools of forensic pharmacology and toxicology come into play, much like in the case of drug checking [82]. Unless take at – or in timely context of – the incident urine and blood sampling suffer from the low diagnostic window and are mostly useless. In contrast, high-resolution hair-sampling might provide valuable information over considerable time-spans [83], which also allows to confirm or falsify previous information form anamnesis or testimonials.

5.4 Case study 2: uncovering a medication induced sleep accident

One morning in May, a fifty-year-old woman cased an accident on the highway in commuter traffic. She reported to have nodded off, causing the accident in consequence. She also stated to have taken the sleeping pill Zolpidem and the anti-depressant Trazodone the evening before and an additional antidepressant (Sertraline).

The toxicological examination of blood revealed in fact Zolpidem and Trazodone in therapeutic concentrations and Sertraline in sub-therapeutic concentrations.

Accordingly, the toxicological assessment postulated an improper use of the hypnotic, as Zolpidem was detected at such high concentrations in the morning, despite its short half-life. According the ability to drive (ATD) at the time of the accident was impaired due to improper medication. Accordingly, the road safety authorities ordered for a full traffic medical assessment including a traffic medical examination at level 4.

Here, the women reported to have started taking Trazodone two years prior to the accident as she had developed sleeping problems due top psychosocial problems. Trazodone and Sertraline had been prescribed by her psychiatrist. Additionally, her practitioner had prescribed Zolpidem from time to time. She reported to have taken Zolpidem only rarely, as she had gotten to know of its addictive potential. At the time of the examination, she had ceased to take Zolpidem already for a period. She explained the situation and the resulting accident by accidentally mixing up Zolpidem and Sertraline.

A routine laboratory set for drugs was ordered, In addition, a segmented hair analysis was performed to confirm discontinuation of Zolpidem use.

Status: The patient presented herself in good general condition, cardiopulmonally compensated, no neurological defects, and psych status after MADP inconspicuous/nondescript.

Therapy at exam: Trazodone, Sertraline.

Routine Laboratory:

Urine: Tetrahydrocannabinol (THC), Cocaine, Methadone, Benzodiazepines, Amphetamine, Methamphetamine, Opiates, Barbiturates, Ecstasy, Buprenorphine, Zolpidem, Tramadol, Fentanyl, Ketamine, MDA, Methaqualone, Methylphenidate, Oxycodone, Phencyclidine, Propoxyphene, Spice/K2, Zaleplon: negative, **Trazodone, tricyclic anti-depressants: positive.**

Hair Analysis Results: (Benzodiazepins und Z-Drugs):

1. Segment: ca. 3 cm (proximal, younger, estimated July–September): Zolpidem 49 pg./mg

2. Segment: ca. 2 cm (distal, older, estimated April–June): Zolpidem 120 pg./mg

In all, anamnestic and laboratory information was sufficient to conclude, that there was no continued medication ab- or misused. The information supported the patient's explanation of a singular medication mistake. The patient was compliant and adherent. The MMR's are given and the fitness to drive could be affirmed.

6. Concluding summary

By way of data form so-called "developed" countries we illustrate a striking prevalence of and, subsequently, an imminent threat for traffic safety by sleep-related disorders. In line with the ambition to minimize fatalities, Switzerland approaches mitigating such (and other medical) threats by defining medical minimum requirements for a driving license. Regular or incidence-related control of these requirements in a highly structured process in traffic medicine reflects one possible strategy that is logically consistent with highly regulated health care, administration and society in general. However, the threat form sleepy driving is universal and fundamentally independent of "development" or location. Thus, consolidated expert advice depends largely on facilitated exchange of unequivocal information, potentially even at the danger of oversimplification. In this line, we argue for a more consistent use of the term "sleepiness" and its signs. We furthermore suggest a more consistent use of standardized measurements (MWT) to detect excessive (or existent) daytime sleepiness (EDS) as the most relevant consequence of sleep conditions met most often in traffic medicine (OSAS, narcolepsy, substance induced EDS). It is often not strikingly bizarre sleep disorders but rather unidentified ones that present the highest risks for traffic. Thus, we inform about simple but clear signs of sleepiness. This is to sensitize both practitioners and experts. These should have an open eye a.) for the interplay between seemingly unrelated conditions potentially leading to EDS affecting the fitness to drive and b.) for the relevance of uncontrolled, uninformed and unintentional substance ab- and misuse affecting the ability to drive. In particular, the latter aspect depends not only on a particular legal and administrative framework's setup, but also on the general or individual attitude in society.

Acknowledgements

This work was supported from the Emma-Louise-Kessler-Fund, a generous donation to the Institute of legal medicine by the late Emma Louise Kessler. The manuscript was written within the project grant Sim_1, which was granted to SL. SL was paid from these project funds.

Conflict of interest

The authors declare to have no conflicts of interest.

Author details

Stefan Lakämper† and Kristina Keller*†
University of Zurich, Institute for Legal Medicine, Traffic Medicine, Zürich, Switzerland

*Address all correspondence to: kristina.keller@irm.uzh.ch

† These authors contributed equally to this work.

References

[1] ASTRA. Strassenverkehrsunfall-Statistik. 2019.

[2] Institute USII. Facts + Statistics: drowsy driving New York, USA: Insurance Information Institute 2020 [Available from: https://www.iii.org/fact-statistic/facts-statistics-drowsy-driving.

[3] Analysis NsNCfSa. Overview of motor vehicle crashes in 2019 (Traffic Safety Facts Research Note. Report No. DOT HS 813 060). 2020, December

[4] bfu. Müdigkeit am Steuer - Wach ans Ziel In: Unfallverhütung b-Bf, editor. Bern: bfu; 2011.

[5] Mathis J, Seeger R, Ewert U. Excessive daytime sleepiness, crashes and driving capability. Schweizer Archiv für Neurologie und Psychiatrie. 2003;154(7):329-38.

[6] Laube I, Seeger R, Russi EW, Bloch KE. Accidents related to sleepiness: review of medical causes and prevention with special reference to Switzerland. Schweiz Med Wochenschr. 1998;128(40):1487-99.

[7] Brennan R. Tiredness killing Aussies with more than 3000 deaths a year linked to lack of sleep. The Daily Telegraphy 2017.

[8] Control USCfD. Sleep and Sleep Disorders Washington, USA: U.S. Centre for Disease Control; 2020

[9] Prevention CfDC. Drowsy driving-19 states and the District of Columbia, 2009-2010. MMWR Morbidity and mortality weekly report. 2013;61(51-52):1033-7.

[10] Klauer SG, Dingus TA, Neale VL, Sudweeks JD, Ramsey DJ. The impact of driver inattention on near-crash/crash risk: An analysis using the 100-car naturalistic driving study data. 2006.

[11] Tefft BC. Prevalence of motor vehicle crashes involving drowsy drivers, United States, 2009-2013: Citeseer; 2014.

[12] Altevogt BM, Colten HR. Sleep disorders and sleep deprivation: an unmet public health problem2006.

[13] Mathis J, Schreier D, Pfäffli M. Tagesschläfrigkeit und Strassenverkehr: Stämpfli Verlag AG Bern; 2016.

[14] Dassanayake T, Michie P, Carter G, Jones A. Effects of benzodiazepines, antidepressants and opioids on driving. Drug safety. 2011;34(2):125-56.

[15] Strassenverkehrsgesetz.

[16] Verordnung über die Zulassung von Personen und Fahrzeugen zum Strassenverkehr (Verkehrszulassungsverordnung, VZV).

[17] Lange A, Keller K, Lakämper S. Buckle up! Rechtsmedizin. 2020;30(5): 283-291. DOI: 10.1007/s00194-020-00418-9

[18] Mosimann U, Bächli-Biétry J, Boll J, Bopp-Kistler I, Donati F, Kressig R, et al. Konsensusempfehlungen zur Beurteilung der medizinischen Mindestanforderungen für Fahreignung bei kognitiver Beeinträchtigung. Praxis. 2012;101(7):451-64.

[19] Leitfaden Fahreignung 2020, (2020).

[20] Krenn N, Keller K. Bewusstseinsstörung am Steuer – nützliche anamnestische Angaben und weiterführende Untersuchungen zur Unterstützung bei zur Beurteilung der Fahrfähigkeit und Fahreignung. Praxis 2021;110 (3):1-6. DOI: https://doi.org/10.1024/1661-8157/a003627

[21] Seeger R, Schaffhauser R. Blackout am Steuer. Verkehrsmedizinische

Betrachtung einer häufig folgenträchtigen Einlassung: Universität St. Gallen; 2010.

[22] Dinges DF. An overview of sleepiness and accidents. Journal of sleep research. 1995;4:4-14.

[23] Hildebrandt G, Moser M, Lehofer M. Chronobiologie und Chronomedizin–kurzgefaßtes Lehr-und Arbeitsbuch1998.

[24] Mathis J, Kohler M, Hemmeter U-M, Seeger R, editors. Fahreignung bei Tagesschläfrigkeit. Swiss medical forum; 2017: EMH Schweizerischer Ärzteverlag AG.

[25] Reppert SM, Weaver DR. Coordination of circadian timing in mammals. Nature. 2002;418(6901): 935-941. DOI: 10.1038/nature00965

[26] Isojima Y, Nakajima M, Ukai H, Fujishima H, Yamada RG, Masumoto K-h, et al. CKIε/δ-dependent phosphorylation is a temperature-insensitive, period-determining process in the mammalian circadian clock. Proceedings of the National Academy of Sciences. 2009;106(37): 15744-15749. DOI: 10.1073/pnas.0908733106

[27] Shen J, Barbera J, Shapiro CM. Distinguishing sleepiness and fatigue: focus on definition and measurement. Sleep Medicine Reviews. 2006;10(1): 63-76. DOI: https://doi.org/10.1016/j.smrv.2005.05.004

[28] Arand D, Bonnet M, Hurwitz T, Mitler M, Rosa R, Sangal RB. The clinical use of the MSLT and MWT. Sleep. 2005;28(1):123-144. DOI: 10.1093/sleep/28.1.123

[29] Dietmann A, Maire M, Bargiotas P, Mathis J, Auer R, Bassetti CL. Tagesschläfrigkeit, Hypersomnie oder Tagesmüdigkeit? Swiss medical forum. 2019:319-324.

[30] Wikipedia. International Classification of Sleep Disorders: Wikipedia; 2021 [updated 31.01.2021.

[31] American Academy of Sleep M. International classification of sleep disorders2014.

[32] Sateia MJ. International Classification of Sleep Disorders-Third Edition. Chest. 2014;146(5):1387-94. DOI: https://doi.org/10.1378/chest.14-0970

[33] Johns MW. Sleep propensity varies with behaviour and the situation in which it is measured: the concept of somnificity. J Sleep Res. 2002;11(1):61-67. DOI: 10.1046/j.1365-2869.2002.00274.x

[34] Pacheco D. Excessive Sleepiness - What it is, its causes and consequences, and how it's diagnosed and treated 2021 [Available from: https://www.sleepfoundation.org/excessive-sleepiness.

[35] Stuck BA, Maurer JT, Schlarb AA, Schredl M, Weeß H-G. Praxis der Schlafmedizin: Diagnostik, Differenzial diagnostik und Therapie bei Erwachsenen und Kindern: Springer-Verlag; 2017.

[36] Finsterer J, Mahjoub SZ. Fatigue in Healthy and Diseased Individuals. American Journal of Hospice and Palliative Medicine®. 2014;31(5): 562-75. DOI: 10.1177/1049909113494748

[37] Kolla BP, He J-P, Mansukhani MP, Frye MA, Merikangas K. Excessive sleepiness and associated symptoms in the U.S. adult population: prevalence, correlates, and comorbidity. Sleep Health. 2020;6(1):79-87. DOI: https://doi.org/10.1016/j.sleh.2019.09.004

[38] Foundation NS. Yearly Sleep in America Poll collection Washington 2021 [Available from: https://www.sleephealthjournal.org/content/sleepinamerica.

[39] Foundation NS. 2008 SLEEP IN AMERICA POLL - SUMMARY OF

FINDINGS. Washington National Sleep Foundation; 2008 01.04.2028.

[40] SWANSON LM, ARNEDT JT, ROSEKIND MR, BELENKY G, BALKIN TJ, DRAKE C. Sleep disorders and work performance: findings from the 2008 National Sleep Foundation Sleep in America poll. Journal of Sleep Research. 2011;20(3):487-94. DOI: https://doi.org/10.1111/j.1365-2869.2010.00890.x

[41] Slater G, Steier J. Excessive daytime sleepiness in sleep disorders. J Thorac Dis. 2012;4(6):608-616. DOI: 10.3978/j.issn.2072-1439.2012.10.07

[42] Hobson JA, Silvestri R. Sleep Disorders. In: Aminoff MJ, Daroff RB, editors. Encyclopedia of the Neurological Sciences. New York: Academic Press; 2003. p. 287-292.

[43] Drake C, Gumenyuk V, Roth T, Howard R. Effects of armodafinil on simulated driving and alertness in shift work disorder. Sleep. 2014;37(12): 1987-1994. DOI: 10.5665/sleep.4256

[44] Philip P, Chaufton C, Taillard J, Capelli A, Coste O, Leger D, et al. Modafinil improves real driving performance in patients with hypersomnia: a randomized double-blind placebo-controlled crossover clinical trial. Sleep. 2014;37(3):483-7.

[45] Billiard M. Hypersomnias Other than Narcolepsy: Differential Diagnosis. Narcolepsy: Springer; 2016. p. 129-146.

[46] Carley DW, Prasad B, Reid KJ, Malkani R, Attarian H, Abbott SM, et al. Pharmacotherapy of Apnea by Cannabimimetic Enhancement, the PACE Clinical Trial: Effects of Dronabinol in Obstructive Sleep Apnea. Sleep. 2018;41(1). DOI: 10.1093/sleep/zsx184

[47] Hug M, Lakämper S, Keller K, Wick R. Tagesschläfrigkeit bei Patienten mit Restless-Legs-Syndrom: Risikofaktor für Verkehrsunfälle? Praxis. 2018;107(24):1319-1323. DOI: 10.1024/1661-8157/a003131

[48] Maffli E. Einnahmemuster von Schlaf-und Beruhi-gungsmitteln in der Allgemeinbevölkerung. Schweizerische Ärztezeitung. 2001;82(47):2479-82.

[49] Steiger A, Weber F, Benkert O. Medikamente zur Behandlung von Schlafstörungen. In: Benkert O, Hippius H, editors. Kompendium der Psychiatrischen Pharmakotherapie. Berlin, Heidelberg: Springer Berlin Heidelberg; 2019. p. 555-640.

[50] Lim ZW, Wang ID, Liu F-C, Chung C-H, Hu J-M, Tsai P-Y, et al. Non-apnea sleep disorder and its risk for all kinds of injuries: A 14-year follow-up for a nationwide population-based retrospective study. Medicine (Baltimore). 2021;100(8):e24766-e. DOI: 10.1097/MD.0000000000024766

[51] Psychomotor disorders [Available from: https://www.sciencedirect.com/topics/neuroscience/psychomotor-d isorder.

[52] Driving and Parkinson's Disease [Available from: https://www.parkinson.org/Living-with-Parkinsons/Managing-Parkinsons/Activities-of-Daily-Living/Driving.

[53] Daniela Schuler AT, Nathalie Buscher, Paul Camenzind,. Psychische Gesundheit in der Schweiz, Monitoring 2016. Neuchâtel, Switzerland: Schweizerisches Gesundheitsobservatorium (Obsan); 2016.

[54] Keller K. Fahrfähigkeit und Fahreignung unter Behandlung mit Psychopharmaka/Schlafmitteln. Praxis. 2018;107(5):245-51.

[55] Verster JC, Roth T. Gender differences in highway driving performance after administration of

sleep medication: a review of the literature. Traffic Inj Prev. 2012;13(3): 286-292. DOI: 10.1080/15389588.2011.652751

[56] Daniela Schuler AT, Claudio Peter. Psychische Gesundheit in der Schweiz, Monitoring 2020. Neuchâtel, Switzerland: Schweizerisches Gesundheitsobservatorium (Obsan); 2020.

[57] de Gier JJ, Alvarez FJ, Mercier-Guyon C, Verstraete AG. Prescribing and dispensing guidelines for medicinal drugs affecting driving performance. Drugs, driving and traffic safety: Springer; 2009. p. 121-34.

[58] Álvarez González FJ, Gómez Talegón T, Fierro I. Establishment of framework for classification/categorisation and labelling of medicinal drugs and driving. 2011.

[59] ICADST Drug list.

[60] CATEGORIZATION SYSTEM FOR MEDICINAL DRUGS AFFECTING DRIVING PERFORMANCE.

[61] Schulz H, Salzarulo P. The Development of Sleep Medicine: A Historical Sketch. J Clin Sleep Med. 2016;12(7):1041-1052. DOI: 10.5664/jcsm.5946

[62] Shepard JW, Jr., Buysse DJ, Chesson AL, Jr., Dement WC, Goldberg R, Guilleminault C, et al. History of the development of sleep medicine in the United States. J Clin Sleep Med. 2005;1(1):61-82.

[63] Berger H. Ueber das Elektroenkephalogramm des Menschen./Arch. Psychiat. 1929.

[64] Loomis AL, Harvey EN, Hobart GA. Cerebral states during sleep, as studied by human brain potentials. Journal of experimental psychology. 1937;21(2):127.

[65] Aserinsky E, Kleitman N. Regularly occurring periods of eye motility, and concomitant phenomena, during sleep. Science. 1953;118(3062):273-274. DOI: 10.1126/science.118.3062.273

[66] Doghramji K. Melatonin and Its Receptors: A New Class of Sleep-Promoting Agents. Journal of Clinical Sleep Medicine. 2007;3(5 suppl):S17-S23. DOI: doi:10.5664/jcsm.26932

[67] Pilorz V, Tam SKE, Hughes S, Pothecary CA, Jagannath A, Hankins MW, et al. Melanopsin Regulates Both Sleep-Promoting and Arousal-Promoting Responses to Light. PLOS Biology. 2016;14(6):e1002482. DOI: 10.1371/journal.pbio.1002482

[68] Ohler N. Blitzed: Drugs in Nazi Germany: Penguin UK; 2016.

[69] Gunja N. In the Zzz zone: the effects of Z-drugs on human performance and driving. J Med Toxicol. 2013;9(2): 163-171. DOI: 10.1007/s13181-013-0294-y

[70] Nonbenzodiazepine [Available from: https://en.wikipedia.org/wiki/Nonbenzodiazepine.

[71] Mets MA, de Vries JM, de Senerpont Domis LM, Volkerts ER, Olivier B, Verster JC. Next-day effects of ramelteon (8 mg), zopiclone (7.5 mg), and placebo on highway driving performance, memory functioning, psychomotor performance, and mood in healthy adult subjects. Sleep. 2011;34 (10):1327-1334. DOI: 10.5665/sleep.1272

[72] Iwata M, Iwamoto K, Kawano N, Kawaue T, Ozaki N. Evaluation method regarding the effect of psychotropic drugs on driving performance: A literature review. Psychiatry and Clinical Neurosciences. 2018;72(10):747-73. DOI: https://doi.org/10.1111/pcn.12734

[73] Vermeeren A, Vets E, Vuurman EFPM, Van Oers ACM,

Jongen S, Laethem T, et al. On-the-road driving performance the morning after bedtime use of suvorexant 15 and 30 mg in healthy elderly. Psychopharmacology (Berl). 2016;233(18):3341-3351. DOI: 10.1007/s00213-016-4375-x

[74] McElroy H, O'Leary B, Adena M, Campbell R, Tahami Monfared AA, Meier G. Comparison of the effect of lemborexant and other insomnia treatments on driving performance: a systematic review and meta-analysis. SLEEP Advances. 2021. DOI: 10.1093/sleepadvances/zpab010

[75] Miyata A, Iwamoto K, Kawano N, Kohmura K, Yamamoto M, Aleksic B, et al. The effects of acute treatment with ramelteon, triazolam, and placebo on driving performance, cognitive function, and equilibrium function in healthy volunteers. Psychopharmacology (Berl). 2015;232 (12):2127-2137. DOI: 10.1007/s00213-014-3843-4

[76] Verster JC, Veldhuijzen DS, Volkerts ER. Residual effects of sleep medication on driving ability. Sleep medicine reviews. 2004;8(4):309-25.

[77] Louwerens JW, Brookhuis KA, O'hanlon JF. The effects of the antidepressants oxaprotiline, mianserin, amitryptiline and doxepin upon actual driving performance 1984.

[78] Katwala J, Kumar AK, Sejpal JJ, Terrence M, Mishra M. Therapeutic rationale for low dose doxepin in insomnia patients. Asian Pac J Trop Dis. 2013;3(4):331-336. DOI: 10.1016/S2222-1808(13)60080-8

[79] Suhner A, Schlagenhauf P, Tschopp A, Hauri-Bionda R, Friedrich-Koch A, Steffen R. Impact of melatonin on driving performance. Journal of travel medicine. 1998;5(1):7-13.

[80] Otmani S, Demazieres A, Staner C, Jacob N, Nir T, Zisapel N, et al. Effects of prolonged-release melatonin, zolpidem, and their combination on psychomotor functions, memory recall, and driving skills in healthy middle aged and elderly volunteers. Human Psychopharmacology: Clinical and Experimental. 2008;23(8):693-705.

[81] Graw P, Werth E, Kräuchi K, Gutzwiller F, Cajochen C, Wirz-Justice A. Early morning melatonin administration impairs psychomotor vigilance. Behavioural brain research. 2001;121(1-2):167-72.

[82] Jones AW, Musshoff F, Kraemer T, Schwaninger AE, Gerostamoulos D, Drummer OH, et al. Toxicology of Specific Substances. Handbook of Forensic Medicine2014. p. 900-993.

[83] Madry MM, Kraemer T, Baumgartner MR. Large scale consumption monitoring of benzodiazepines and z-drugs by hair analysis. Journal of pharmaceutical and biomedical analysis. 2020;183:113151.

Chapter 8

Circadian Rhythm Disorders

Ajay Sampat and Armand Ryden

Abstract

Circadian rhythm disorders are a group of sleep conditions that involve a misalignment of an individual's internal timekeeping system with that of one's desired sleep-wake time. This desynchrony can compromise sleep health as well as the functioning of other organ system, and significantly diminish one's quality of life. There are six well-defined circadian rhythm disorders that can be classified as either intrinsic or extrinsic, based on the underlying factors that contribute to the condition. Intrinsic circadian disorders include the following: 1) advanced sleep-wake phase disorder, 2) delayed sleep-wake phase disorder, 3) irregular sleep-wake rhythm disorder, and 4) non-24-hour sleep-wake rhythm disorder. The two circadian disorders caused by external factors include 1) shift work disorder, and 2) jet lag disorder, both of which are due to behaviorally mediated misalignments of circadian system. This chapter serves to summarize these disorders, guide clinicians towards screening and evaluation of these conditions, and introduce basic treatment strategies that can be applied by non-sleep medicine clinicians.

Keywords: circadian rhythm disorder, advanced sleep–wake phase disorder, delayed sleep–wake phase disorder, irregular sleep–wake rhythm disorder, non-24-hour sleep–wake rhythm disorder, shift work disorder, jet lag disorder, melatonin, phototherapy

1. Introduction: what every clinician needs to know

The intrinsic circadian system synchronizes basic physiologic functions such as temperature regulation, appetite, and hormonal homeostasis and is responsible for the stable sleep and wake states that occur at regular times with respect to day and night. The term circadian derives from the Latin words "circa," meaning approximately, and "diem," meaning day, which emphasize that the intrinsic cycle is usually not exactly 24 hours in length [1]. The average circadian cycle length is generally 24.2 hours, which means that the cycle always requires entrainment to the environment because the day is exactly 24 hours long. Light is the most potent mechanism of entrainment, but meals and exercise also have an impact on entrainment [1–3]. Dysynchrony between a person's internal circadian system and their desired wake and sleep periods can lead to one of 6 different types of circadian rhythm sleep–wake disorders (CRSWDs). These disorders can present clinically with symptoms of insomnia and/or excessive daytime sleepiness, along with impairments in cognitive, emotional, and social functioning. A key feature of these conditions is that re-alignment of the intrinsic circadian period to the desired circadian period leads to resolution of symptoms.

CRSWDs may be due to a primary problem with the circadian system, such as altered sensitivity of the circadian system to light, and genetic and/or age-related factors that disrupt the intrinsic period of the system.

The diagnosis of CRSWDs can be difficult, due to the overlapping symptoms with other sleep disorders and medical conditions. Recognizing consistent patterns in abnormal sleep schedules is key to helping differentiate CRSWDs from other disorders. CRSWDs are primarily clinical diagnoses and use of a detailed sleep diary is an important part of the evaluation. Other objective measures such as actigraphy and melatonin measurements can supplement information obtained from the patient's history [4]. Polysomnography is usually not indicated unless there is a suspicion for a comorbid sleep disorder, such as a sleep-related breathing disorder.

Management of circadian rhythm sleep–wake disorders involves a combination of behavioral interventions, light therapy, and timed melatonin therapy. Treatment is individualized to the specific circadian rhythm sleep–wake disorder [5]. The goal of therapy is to gradually realign the patient's sleep and wake times with the desired schedule. The timing of light and melatonin therapies is critical to determining their biologic effects. The key biologic markers are the dim light melatonin onset (DLMO), which typically occurs approximately two hours prior to habitual sleeptime, and the core body temperature minimum (CBT-min), which typically occurs 2-3 hours prior to habitual wake up time. Exposure to light prior to the body temperature minimum will cause the circadian rhythm to delay (i.e. the next night, there will be a tendency to go to bed and wake up later). Light exposure after the core body temperature minimum will cause the circadian system to advance (i.e. the next night, there will be a tendency to go to bed and to wake up earlier). The effect of light is most potent when it is in the blue spectrum and administered close to the CBT-min. Melatonin has the opposite phase response relationship that light has; melatonin given prior to the CBT-min will cause the circadian rhythm to advance (i.e., the next night, there will be a tendency to go to bed and wake up earlier) whereas melatonin administration after the CBT-min will cause the circadian system to delay (i.e., the next night, there will be a tendency to go to bed and wake up later).

The International Classification of Sleep Disorders, third edition (ICSD-3), has the following three diagnostic criteria for all circadian rhythm sleep–wake disorders [6]:

1. A disrupted sleep–wake pattern, thought to be due to misalignment or malfunction of the circadian system;

2. A complaint of insomnia, excessive sleepiness, or both;

3. Suboptimal performance in an important area of functioning (e.g. occupation, education, social life, mental or physical life).

2. Classification of the circadian rhythm sleep-wake disorders

Intrinsic CRSWDs include the following: 1) advanced sleep–wake phase disorder (extreme early bird), 2) delayed sleep–wake phase disorder (extreme night owl), 3) non-24-hour sleep–wake rhythm disorder (drifting circadian rhythm), and 4) irregular sleep–wake rhythm disorder (no rhythm). The two circadian disorders caused by extrinsic factors are 1) shift work disorder and 2) jet lag disorder, both of which are due to behaviorally mediated misalignments of circadian system.

3. Are you sure your patient has a circadian rhythm sleep-wake disorder? What should you expect to find?

Circadian rhythm disorders can result in clinically significant symptoms of insomnia, excessive daytime sleepiness, and cognitive impairment. In addition, a drastic misalignment of one's circadian clock with societal norms can often have implications for one's emotional well-being and social functioning. There are 6 major categories of circadian rhythm sleep–wake disorders which are grouped based on patterns of sleep time:

3.1 Advanced sleep–wake phase disorder (ASWPD)

ICSD-3 Diagnostic Criteria [6]:

1. An advance (early timing) in the phase of the major sleep episode in relation to the desired or required sleep time and wake-up time, (i.e. the patient feels sleepy too early and wakes up too early).

2. Symptoms are present for at least three months.

3. When the patient sleeps of his/her own accord, sleep quality and duration are improved with a consistent but advanced timing of the major sleep episode.

4. Sleep log and, whenever possible, actigraphy monitoring for at least seven days show a stable advance in sleep period. Both work/school days and free days must be included during the actigraphy monitoring period.

5. The patient's symptoms are not better explained by another current sleep, medical, neurological disorder or mental disorder.

Clinical Characteristics: ASWPD is an intrinsic defect of the circadian system in which sleep duration and quality are normal, but where sleep and wake up times are earlier than desired or socially acceptable. Generally, the intrinsic circadian rhythm period is actually shorter than normal.

Patients with ASWPD often report that they are unable to stay awake past 7 PM and tend to wake up around 2-5 AM. If a patient is able to set their own schedule they will obtain adequate sleep and feel refreshed in the morning. However, since due to social obligations they often stay up later than naturally desired while still waking early. This can lead to a sleep deficit over time that leads to daytime sleepiness.

3.2 Delayed sleep-wake phase disorder (DSWPD)

ICSD-3 Diagnostic Criteria [6]: A delay (late timing) in the phase of the major sleep episode in relation to the desired or required sleep time and wake-up time (i.e. the patient does not feel sleepy at bed time and wakes up too late).

6. The symptoms are present for at least three months.

7. When patients sleep of their own accord, sleep quality and duration are improved with a consistent but delayed timing of the major sleep episode.

8. Sleep log and, whenever possible, actigraphy monitoring for at least seven days show a stable delay in sleep period. Both work/school days and free days must be included during the actigraphy monitoring period.

9. The patient's symptoms are not better explained by another current sleep, medical, neurological disorder or mental disorder

Clinical Characteristics: DSWPD is one of the most common circadian rhythm sleep–wake disorders, often affecting adolescents and young adults when eveningness tendencies are typically the strongest. This is a defect of the circadian system whereby the sleep/wake cycle is misaligned with the patient's desired schedule by more than 2 hours. Individuals go to sleep and wake up at substantially later times than desired, which can lead to social consequences such as chronic tardiness at work or school. Delayed bedtimes (usually between 1 and 6 AM), coupled with early awakenings to meet social/occupational/academic obligations, result in a sleep debt that accumulates over time. There is often a high prevalence of comorbid depression, and higher degrees of circadian misalignment correlate with greater severity of depression.

The intrinsic circadian period is generally longer than normal. DSWPD typically emerges during adolescence and can continue into adulthood.

3.3 Irregular sleep-wake rhythm disorder (ISWRD)

ICSD-3 Diagnostic Criteria [6]:

1. Chronic or recurrent pattern of irregular sleep and wake episodes throughout the 24-hour period.

2. Symptoms are present for at least three months.

3. Sleep log and, whenever possible, actigraphy monitoring for at least seven days, show no major sleep period and multiple irregular sleep bouts (at least three) during a 24-hour period.

4. The patient's symptoms are not better explained by another current sleep, medical, neurological disorder or mental disorder.

Clinical Characteristics: ISWRD is characterized by a temporally disorganized sleep and wake pattern such that there are no clearly defined periods of wake and/or sleep. Multiple sleep and wake periods can occur throughout the day, and usually consist of 3 or more short intervals, approximately 1-4 hours each. The longest period generally occurs in the morning between 2 and 6 AM; however, the distribution of sleep and wake periods can vary per individual. The total sleep duration throughout a 24-hour period is generally normal for the individual's age. Because of the fragmented nature of sleep, individuals can experience frequent napping, excessive daytime sleepiness, and difficulty staying asleep at night.

3.4 Non-24 sleep-wake rhythm disorder (N24SWRD)

ICSD-3 Diagnostic Criteria [6]:

1. History of insomnia, excessive daytime sleepiness, or both, which alternate with asymptomatic episodes, due to misalignment between the 24-hour light–dark cycle and the non-entrained endogenous circadian rhythm of sleep–wake propensity.

2. Symptoms persist over the course of at least three months.

3. Daily sleep logs and actigraphy for at least 14 days, preferably longer for blind persons, show a pattern of sleep and wake times that typically delay each day.

4. The patient's symptoms are not better explained by another current sleep, medical, neurological disorder or mental disorder.

Clinical Characteristics: N24SWD, also known as non-trained rhythm disorder, is characterized by chronic cycles of sleep and wake that are not always synchronized with the 24-hour environment. There is a gradual, but consistent drift of sleep and wake times later into the day. Attempting to maintain a regular sleep–wake schedule can lead to symptoms of excessive daytime sleepiness, chronic fatigue, early morning awakenings and insomnia. These symptoms alternate with days to weeks in which the patient is asymptomatic, owing to the patient's endogenous circadian system coinciding with the external 24-hour cycle. Napping is common, and patients often report impairment of social and occupational functioning due to non-entrained sleep–wake schedule.

N24SWD occurs most often in blind individuals. Onset of symptoms usually occurs in 2nd or 3rd decade of life, and men are disproportionally affected compared to women at a ratio of >2: 1 [7].

3.5 Shift work sleep-wake disorder (SWD)

ICSD-3 Diagnostic Criteria [6]:

1. Insomnia and/or excessive sleepiness, accompanied by a reduction of total sleep time, which is associated with a recurring work schedule that overlaps with the usual time for sleep.

2. Symptoms are present and associated with the shift work schedule for at least three months.

3. Symptoms cause clinically significant impairment in mental, physical, social, occupational, education, or other important areas of functioning.

4. Sleep log and, whenever possible, actigraphy monitoring for at least 14 days (work and free days) demonstrate a disturbed sleep and wake pattern.

5. The patient's symptoms are not better explained by another current sleep, medical, neurological disorder or mental disorder.

Clinical Characteristics: Individuals who work night shift experience difficulty with sleep and alertness at desired times, and are at greater risk for the variety of adverse health outcomes associated with poor sleep. Shift workers generally report 30-90 minutes less sleep compared to those not working shifts, and their sleep quality tends to be more fragmented and of poorer quality. Shift workers also experience difficulty falling and staying asleep, with as many as 20% of shift workers having clinically significant insomnia [8]. During waking hours, night shift workers are more prone to increased sleepiness, decreased neurocognitive function and more significant changes to mood than their non-night shift counterparts.

3.6 Jet lag disorder (JLD)

ICSD-3 Diagnostic Criteria [6]:

1. Insomnia or excessive daytime sleepiness associated with a reduction of total sleep time coinciding with jet travel across at least two time zones

2. Impaired daytime function, general fatigue, or somatic symptoms that begin within two days of travel

3. The sleep disturbance cannot be explained by another disorder.

Clinical Characteristics: JLD occurs when an individual travels through time zones faster that the endogenous circadian rhythm can adjust, resulting in desynchrony between the external light–dark cycle and one's internal clock. Symptoms of JLD include difficulty falling and staying asleep, excessive daytime sleepiness, generalized fatigue, impaired daytime performance, and various somatic symptoms (most commonly gastrointestinal) that begin 1 to 2 days post-travel [8].

In addition to number of time zones traveled, the severity of jet lag is affected by the direction of travel. Eastward travel leads to more difficulty with falling asleep and is more difficult to adjust to, while westward travel is more disruptive to sleep maintenance.

4. How and/or why did the patient develop a circadian rhythm sleep-wake disorder? Which individuals are of greatest risk of developing a circadian rhythm sleep-wake disorder?

4.1 Advanced sleep-wake phase disorder (ASWPD)

Genetic studies have shown possible links to mutations in the *PER2* and *CSNK1D* clock genes, both of which are inherited in autosomal dominant pattern [2, 3]. There is an estimated 1% prevalence, with males and females being equally affected. Older adults are more likely to have advanced tendencies. Other contributing factors include decreased responsiveness to evening light, and increased responsiveness to morning light, both of which can shift the sleep–wake cycle earlier than desired.

4.2 Delayed sleep–wake phase disorder (DSWPD)

The pathophysiology of DSWPD is multifactorial [2, 3] l. It is hypothesized that certain exogenous factors, such as increased exposure to evening light and greater sensitivity to evening light may play a role in development of DSWPD. Genetic factors may play a role, but their exact contribution is less understood than is the case for ASWPD.

DSWPD typically emerges during adolescence and can continue into adulthood. Males and females seem to be affected equally. Peak age appears to be 21 years old in males and 17 years old in females. There is a large variability in its reported prevalence, with population study estimates ranging from <1% up to 10% [1–3]. Patients with hepatic cirrhosis are also affected at much higher rates (33%).

4.3 Irregular sleep-wake rhythm disorder (ISWRD)

ISWRD is most commonly seen in individuals with neurodegenerative conditions, particularly those with Alzheimer's disease and late-afternoon sundowning [1–3]. It is also more common in those with traumatic brain injury, in children with developmental delay, in patients with schizophrenia, and particularly in patients who are institutionalized. It is hypothesized that intrinsic circadian dysfunction, coupled with decreased exposure to external synchronizing agents such as light and social activity, are factors in ISWRD.

4.4 Non-24 sleep-wake rhythm disorder (N24SWRD)

The etiology of N24SWD is related to disruption of the portion of the circadian system responsible for capturing photic stimuli in the retina. Pathologies that lead to vision loss often but not necessarily impact this system. Thus, N24SWD occurs most often in blind individuals, with reports of 50% of blind patients diagnosed with N24SWD and up to 70% of blind individuals having symptoms of chronic sleep disturbance [2, 3, 7]. Men are disproportionally affected compared to women at a ratio of >2:1. N24SWD is rare, but has been reported, in sighted individuals. In sighted individuals, N24SWD is thought to be a severe form of delayed sleep phase disorder where entrainment to light can no longer be effective [7].

4.5 Shift work sleep-wake disorder (SWD)

The mechanism behind SWD is thought to be governed by disruptions of 2 physiologic processes [1–3]. The first is related to one's homeostatic drive for sleep, which increases throughout wakefulness. The second is one's intrinsic rhythmic oscillations for sleep and wake periods, which is governed by the circadian pacemaker. This latter process is calibrated by environmental clues such as light. Both the homeostatic process and the circadian process are disrupted in SWD.

Individuals at greatest risk for SWD are those that work rotating night shifts, rather than permanent night shifts, because they are never able to adapt to a stable sleep–wake pattern [8]. In addition, those with other sleep comorbidities can have synergistic effects of sleep disturbance, which lead to symptomatic worsening.

4.6 Jet lag disorder (JLD)

JLD results from desynchrony between the external light–dark cycle and an individual's internal clock when travel across time zones occurs more quickly than the endogenous circadian rhythm can adjust. The prevalence of this condition is poorly defined [8]. Factors that affect jet lag severity include the direction of travel and number of time zones traveled, the person's ability to sleep during travel, individual variations in circadian timing, presence of light cues at destination, and intake of alcohol and caffeine.

5. What diagnostic studies will be helpful in making or excluding the diagnosis of a circadian rhythm sleep-wake disorder? What other diseases can mimic circadian rhythm sleep-wake disorders?

5.1 Advanced sleep-wake phase disorder (ASWPD)

ASWPD is a clinical diagnosis and should be suspected in individuals who have a history of early sleep onset and wake times. It is important to obtain a detailed sleep history that addresses sleep patterns, napping habits, and daytime symptoms of sleepiness, cognitive changes, or mood changes. Targeted questions should be asked about difficulty falling or staying asleep and sleep quality both during the patient's current schedule and during times when he/she has followed the preferred schedule. Obtaining collateral history from a bed partner is often useful.

Patients with suspected ASWPD should keep a sleep log for at least 7 days, preferably 14 days, including both weekdays and weekends (**Figure 1**). Actigraphy is helpful to supplement the sleep diary, especially if the history is unreliable. Melatonin levels, through salivary or plasma sampling, may show early melatonin onset or earlier phase of melatonin metabolite excretion via urinary 6-sulfatoxymelatonin, although these tests are not widely available for clinical purposes [2, 3, 9].

5.2 Delayed sleep-wake phase disorder (DSWPD)

DSWPD is a clinical diagnosis and should be suspected when individuals report consistent bedtime and wake times that are significantly later than social norms. Bedtimes are often more informative than wake times, which are usually dictated by social or work/school obligations. It is also helpful to ask about sleep patterns during weekends, and during unrestricted periods such as vacations, when patients are able to sleep based on their own circadian preference (**Figure 2**). Sleep logs of at least 7 days, including both school/workdays and weekends, are needed to identify specific patterns [9]. It is important to inquire about other social factors, such as caffeine use later in the day, or excessive use of light-emitting devices before bedtime, which can also delay sleep onset.

Wrist actigraphy is another means of obtaining more quantitative data [9]. If the actigraph has a photo sensor it can provide information about the correlation between an individual's light exposure and sleep time. Polysomnography is not typically indicated, unless there is clinical suspicion for another comorbid sleep disorder, such as sleep-disordered breathing. Salivary melatonin assays are available; however, these assays are used primarily as research tools and not for clinical diagnosis.

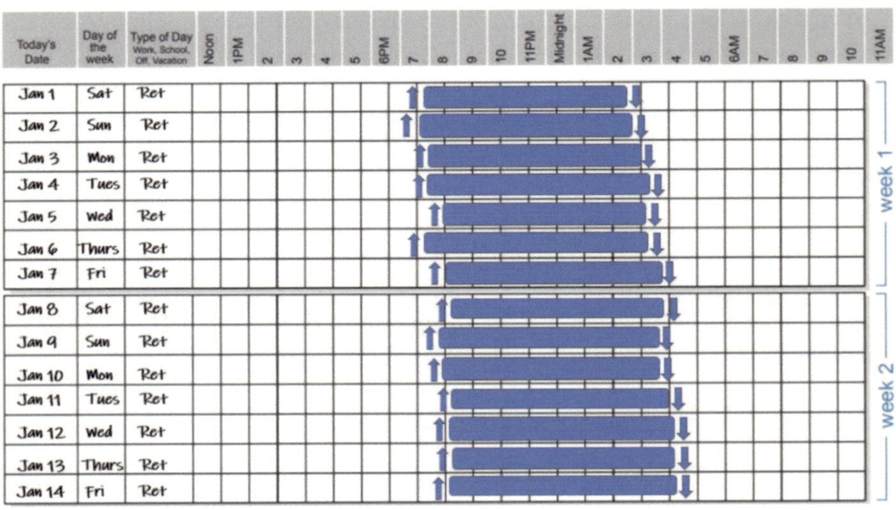

Figure 1.
This 14-day sleep diary of a patient with advanced sleep–wake phase disorder (ASWPD) depicts an early sleep onset (7-8 pm) and early wake time (3-4 am). The total duration of sleep time (shaded box) remains normal at 7-8 hours. Individuals with ASWPD usually do not have symptoms if they are allowed to sleep per their preferred schedule; however, when tasked with staying up later than their usual bedtime, they can have significant difficulty. This circadian rhythm is more prevalent in older adults who may not have the same work or school obligations ("ret" represents "retired") that can contribute to other circadian rhythm disorders, such as delayed sleep–wake phase disorder.

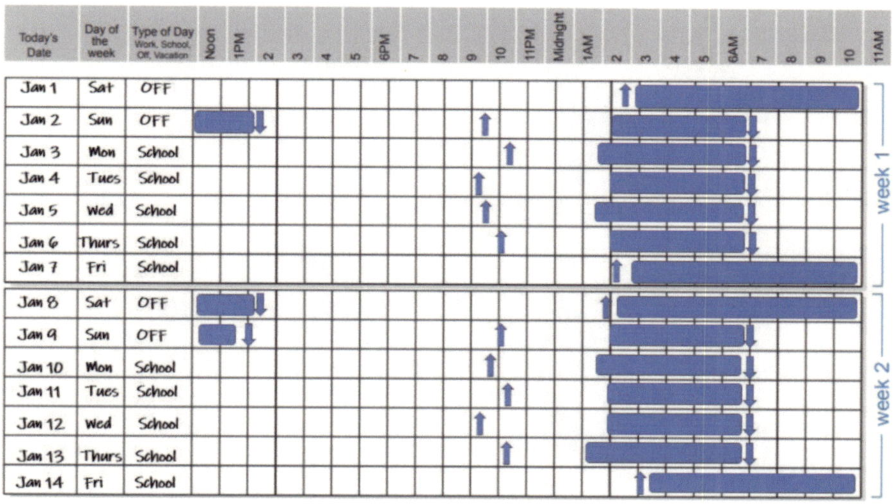

Figure 2.
This 14-day sleep diary of a patient with delayed sleep–wake phase disorder (DSWPD) depicts variable sleep depending on the day of the week. The upwards arrow indicates "time in bed" while the downwards arrow indicates "time out of bed". The shaded area represents sleep time of the patient. For example, in this diagram, the individual goes to bed between 9 and 10 pm on school days but is not able to sleep until 2-3 am. Due to his fixed school start time, he has to get out of bed between 6 and 7 am, leaving only 4-5 hours of sleep time (shaded box). However, on weekends (Friday and Saturday nights), he goes to sleep at his desired time of 2-3 am and wakes up at his desired time between 1 and 2 pm, accounting for a total sleep time of 10-11 hours. This variation in sleep pattern, based on day of the week, is classic for DSWPD, and results in the symptoms described by those with this condition.

5.3 Irregular sleep-wake rhythm disorder (ISWRD)

The diagnosis of ISWRD is made by clinical history, with supplemental information from wrist actigraphy. There must be a reported chronic or recurrent pattern of irregular sleep and wake episodes throughout a 24-hour period, with a minimum of 3 cycles occurring during that time (**Figure 3**). A sleep log, and/or actigraphy must document these cycles for at least 7 days (preferably 14 days), and symptoms must be present for at least 3 months [9].

Polysomnography is not usually indicated, unless there is concern that the sleep disturbance is better explained by another disorder (e.g., a sleep-related breathing disorder).

5.4 Non-24 sleep-wake rhythm disorder (N24SWRD)

Sleep diary and actigraphy are important in confirming a non-entrained sleep pattern and will also show a gradual drift of onset and offset of the sleep–wake rhythm (**Figure 4**). In order to appreciate the drift, this data should be obtained for at least 2 weeks, and symptoms should be present for at least 3 months [9].

Other measurements such as continuous core body temperature or serial measurements of melatonin can be confirmatory as they also exhibit a similarly non-24-hour drifting rhythm. However, these procedures are not required to make the diagnosis of N24SWD.

Attention should be paid to distinguish N24SWD from DSWPD, as these patients can display a similar evening phenotype and up to 25% of N24SWD are often initially misdiagnosed as DSWPD [2, 3, 9].

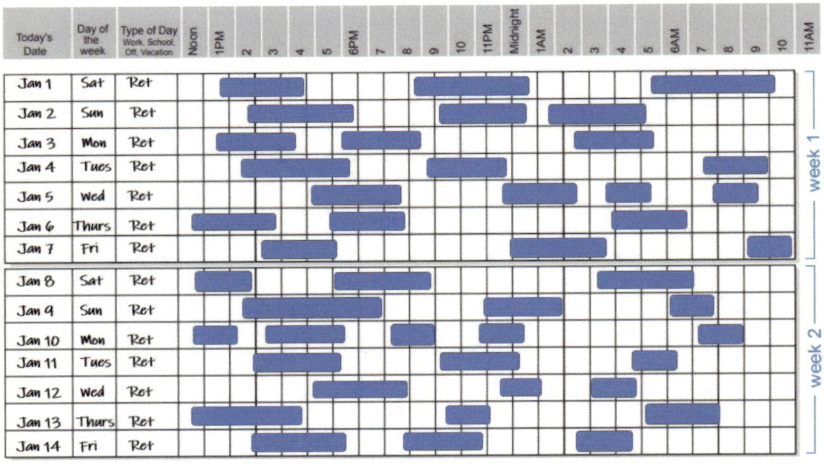

Figure 3.
This 14-day sleep diary of a patient with irregular sleep-wake rhythm disorder (ISWRD) depicts an irregular pattern of sleep throughout each 24-hour period. During each day, there are at least 3 sleep cycles occurring in a recurrent, but irregular fashion. The total sleep duration (shaded box) is usually normal for an individual's age, however there is no clearly defined pattern. This disorder is more prevalent in older individuals and in those with dementia.

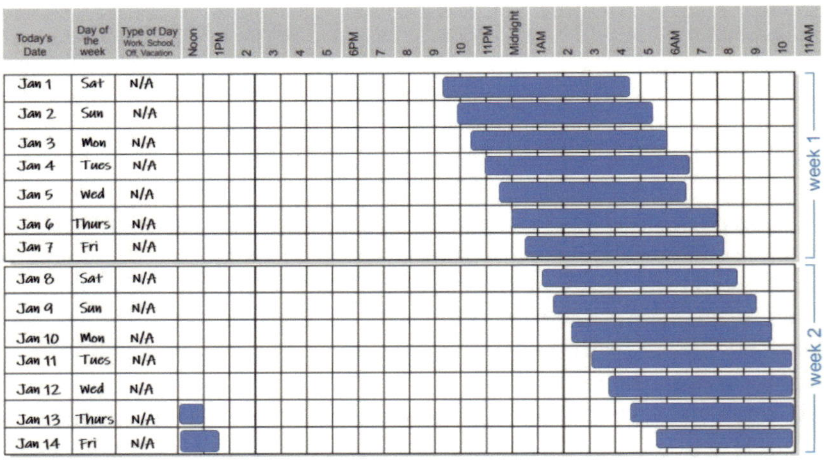

Figure 4.
This 14-day sleep diary of a patient with non-24 sleep–wake phase disorder (N24SWPD) depicts a gradual drift in onset and offset of the sleep duration (shaded box), usually by 30 minutes each day. In order to best appreciate this drift, a sleep diary or actigraphy should be obtained for at least 2 weeks, and ideally more if possible. This circadian rhythm disorder is most prevalent in individuals who are blind.

5.5 Shift work sleep-wake disorder (SWD)

SWD is best assessed through careful sleep history and sleep diary. Particular attention should be paid to a patient's occupation, history with shift work disorder with prior jobs, and impaired task performance at work. Factors specific to the patient's home environment (i.e. lack of dedicated dark space for sleeping, noise levels during the day, etc.) can further reduce the likelihood that the patient can obtain restorative sleep. The clinical history should also inquire about features of other comorbid sleep, medical, and mental disorders. A sleep diary should be obtained for at least 2 weeks and should capture both work and non-work days [9]. Validated questionnaires, such as the Insomnia Severity Index and Epworth Sleepiness Scale, can be used but are not required to diagnose SWD.

Wrist actigraphy, especially when performed with an actigraphy that includes a photosensor, can better quantify sleep duration. There is no need for polysomnography unless there is a clinical suspicion for a comorbid sleep disorder, such as a sleep-related breathing disorder. Melatonin sampling is done in research settings, but is not routinely used in the clinical setting.

5.6 Jet lag disorder (JLD)

Clinical history is the most important tool. The clinician should specifically obtain information about number of time zones crossed and the timeline of symptom occurrence. JLD is often confused with travel fatigue since there are many overlapping symptoms; however, the distinction is that travel fatigue is not dependent on the number of time zones traveled and tends to resolve quicker.

Since JLD is transient, and clinical history is usually clear, there is typically no role for formal diagnostic testing.

6. If you decide the patient has a circadian rhythm sleep-wake disorder, how should the patient be managed?

6.1 Advanced sleep-wake phase disorder (ASWPD)

Bright light therapy in the early evening is the primary treatment for ASWPD, with the goal to delay the circadian phase so it is better aligned to desired sleep and wake times [5, 9]. Patients should use a bright light that filters out ultraviolet rays (2,500 to 10,000 lux) for 1-3 hours per day, starting at the time when they first experience sleepiness in the evening (usually around 7-9 pm). This should be done to gradually delay bedtime by 1-2 hours each day until desired times are met (**Figure 5**).

There is no strong evidence to support pharmacologic therapy in ASWPD. Melatonin in the morning can theoretically shift the clock to a later phase, however the sedating effect of melatonin often limits morning use. Early morning hypnotics to resume sleep can lead to daytime grogginess and hangover effect and thus are generally discouraged.

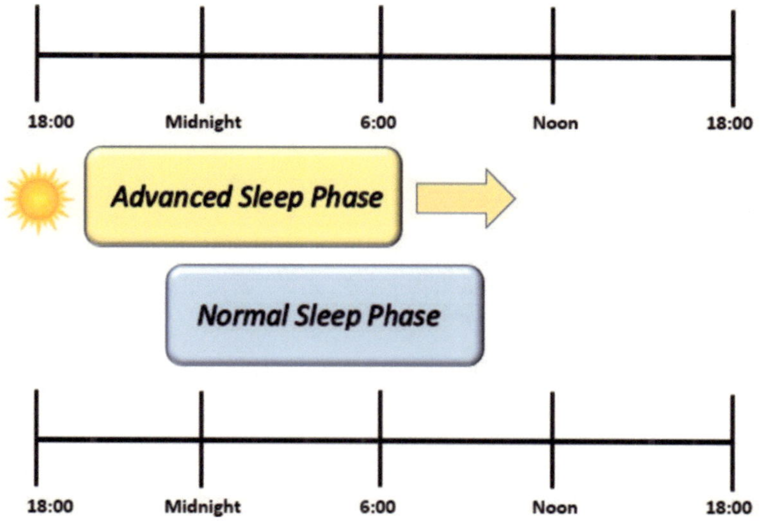

Figure 5.
For individuals with advanced sleep–wake phase disorder (ASWPD), bright light therapy should be given for 1-3 hours per day in the evening starting at the time of sleepiness. This will gradually shift the sleep time until the desired schedule is met.

6.2 Delayed sleep-wake phase disorder (DSWPD)

Management of DSWPD consists of *behavioral modifications* to realign one's circadian system with desired sleep–wake times, and concurrent *melatonin* use and *light* therapy. Easily modifiable behaviors should be targeted first. These behaviors include avoiding daytime naps, eliminating excessive use of caffeine and/or alcohol, reducing stimulating activity, and minimizing light (particularly blue light) exposure 2 hours prior to bedtime.

For those who fail to respond to behavioral therapies alone, timed melatonin can supplement these behavioral modifications. One reasonable approach would be to take melatonin daily, approximately 3-5 hours prior to desired sleep time [5]. Doses may vary from 0.5-5 mg, though it is best to use the lowest effective dose. Melatonin dose and timing can be strategically adjusted based on clinical response. Relapse tends to occur in high rates (80-90%) once melatonin is discontinued [3, 5].

Morning light therapy can be coupled with the above interventions. Commercial light boxes that either contain a broad spectrum of white light or narrow spectrum of blue light (2,000-10,000 lux) should be used every morning between just after typical wake-up time, with gradual advancing of the sleep–wake time until the desired time is reached [5, 9]. Care should be taken to avoid light exposure earlier than 2-3 hours before the habitual wake up time because light prior to the core body temperature minimum may cause further delays in circadian phase (**Figure 6**).

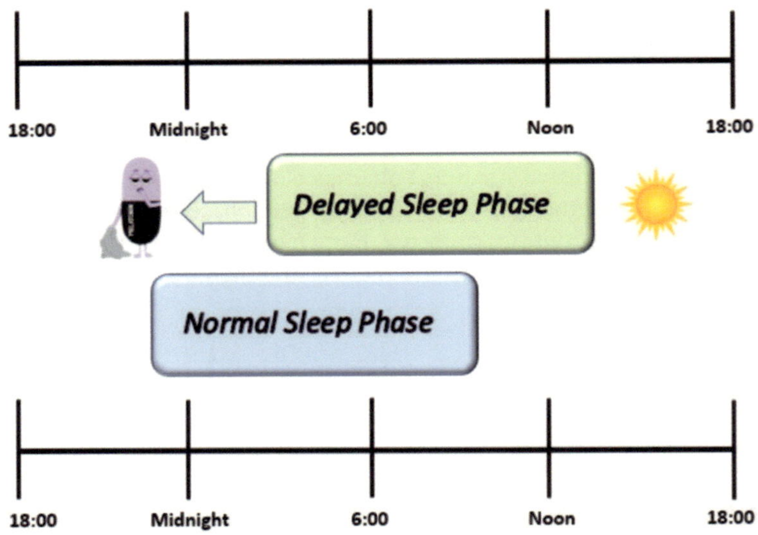

Figure 6.
For individuals with delayed sleep–wake phase disorder (DSWPD), treatment can consist of low-dose melatonin (to be taken ~3-5 hours prior to desired sleep time), along with phototherapy in the morning upon awakening. This combination can cause gradual advancement in sleep phase.

6.3 Irregular sleep–wake rhythm disorder (ISWRD)

Treatment of ISWRD involves using behavioral strategies to restructure an individual's daily routine, and to optimize sleep hygiene to better consolidate sleep times and improve daytime alertness. It is important to create a cognitively enriched and socially interactive environment during the day to maintain alertness and prevent excessive napping. At night, measures should be taken to reduce noise and light, and to prevent sleep disturbances caused by other factors (e.g., nocturia).

Light therapy remains the most effective intervention during the day. Exposure to 3,000-5,000 lux of light for at least 2 hours in the morning has been shown to improve daytime alertness, reduce napping, and consolidate nightly sleep [5].

Melatonin can also be used for management of ISWRD, though positive results with melatonin use are less consistent than with treatment of other CRSWDs. Melatonin doses of 1-5 mg can be used 30 min prior to bedtime to facilitate sleep, and melatonin is more effective if used in conjunction with light therapy [3, 5]. Controlled-release formulation can be more effective than immediate release in this specific patient population with ISWRD.

6.4 Non-24 sleep-wake rhythm disorder (N24SWRD)

Treatment for N24SWD includes attempting to re-synchronize the circadian pacemaker using behavioral approaches and pharmacologic therapy. Education regarding proper sleep hygiene and maintenance of regularly scheduled timing of meals, social activities and physical exercise is important.

Tasimelteon, a melatonin agonist with affinity for the MT1 and MT2 receptors, is Food and Drug Administration (FDA) approved for use in N24SWD [5]. Melatonin can also be used to achieve gradual re-alignment. Higher doses (3-10 mg) may be given 1-2 hours prior to the desired bedtime for the first month. Entrainment usually occurs within 5-10 weeks, after which low-dose melatonin (0.5-1 mg) should be maintained to prevent relapse [5, 7].

Less robust evidence exists for bright light therapy, though it has been shown to be effective in sighted individuals with N24SWD and can be used in the early morning after awakenings.

6.5 Shift work sleep-wake disorder (SWD)

Management of SWD should first start with changes to work schedule, if possible, with adjustments to sleep hygiene. A regular daytime sleep schedule that can be followed, even during non-working days, is recommended to promote stability to the circadian system. This can be organized around an individual's personal schedule, but should ideally incorporate at least a 5 to 6-hour block of uninterrupted sleep. The sleep environment should be optimized to reduce sound, light, unfavorable temperatures and other factors that can interfere with sleep. Light blocking window shades can be used, and a temperature setting between 65 and 70 degrees Fahrenheit is optimal.

While at work, individuals can use continuous exposure to high-intensity light (2,000-10,000 lux) for as little as four 20-minute periods during the first part of the nigh [8] t. Use of blue light-blocking goggles in the morning and general avoidance of morning light help the circadian rhythm remain adapted to the shift work schedule. Additionally, short naps (<45 minutes) prior to the start of the work shift are a low-risk intervention that can be used to promote wakefulness during the shift.

If these behavioral measures fail, medication therapy is the next step. Modafinil (200 mg) and armodafinil (150 mg) are FDA approved for shift work disorder and can be used during the first part of the night [5, 8]. Small doses of caffeine (100-250 mg, equivalent to a small cup of coffee) can also be used during the first part of the night. Short-acting hypnotics such as zolpidem and zaleplon can be used to promote sleep during the daytime; use of hypnotics must be introduced cautiously to prevent nocturnal grogginess (during work hours). Exogenous melatonin 30 min prior to desired bedtime can be used, although the evidence for this is poor [5].

6.6 Jet lag disorder (JLD)

The treatment strategy depends on the length of trip, number of time zones traveled, and direction of travel [9]. Trips less than 3 days are usually too short to create problematic jet lag symptoms. Treatment planning is best done in anticipation of travel.

For eastward travel on trips longer than 3 days and up to 7 time zones, a strategy using timed light exposure and melatonin can help advance the circadian rhythm (making natural bedtime and wake time earlier) to the new time zone. Bright light therapy can be started up to 3 days prior to departure to start the advancing process. Individuals should wake up about 1 hour prior to usual wake-up time and expose themselves to bright light for at least an hour. Upon arrival at destination, strategic light exposure throughout the afternoon and light avoidance during the early morning can help with this circadian realignment. The specific timing of light exposure is based on when the patient's habitual core body temperature minimum (CBT-min) occurs, which is usually 3 hours before habitual wake-up time. Light exposure after the CBT-min causes circadian phase advancement, whereas light exposure before the CBT-min causes a circadian phase delay and is thus counterproductive for eastward travel [8].

Timed melatonin (3-5 mg) taken at the desired destination bedtime can be used concurrently with prescribed light exposure. Melatonin should first be taken on the evening of arrival and continued for up to 5 days. Hypnotics have been used by patients during travel, but these medications can lead to impaired daytime performance, and thus are generally not recommended for management of JLD. Caffeine can help mitigate daytime sleepiness. Other stimulants (e.g. modafinil, armodafinil) can offset daytime sleepiness though these medications are not FDA approved for JLD. For eastward travel that crosses more than 8 time zones, it is often easier to pursue a circadian phase delay, rather than a circadian phase advance, to mitigate symptoms of JLD. This approach generally involves seeking out early morning light at the destination and avoiding light exposure in the afternoon.

Westward travel requires a delay in the circadian rhythm (later bed times and wake times) to adjust to the destination time zone. It is advised to seek bright light before the calculated CBT-min at the destination (based on the home time zone). For example, if one's habitual wake up time in Boston is 8 am Eastern Standard Time (EST), the habitual CBT-min will be at 5 am EST. If that individual travels to Westward to Hawaii (5-hour time zone delay), the CBT-min will occur at midnight EST, thus bright light exposure should be given prior to that time. Melatonin or hypnotics are generally not required in JLD associated with westward travel.

Resources such as www.jetlagrooster.com and the British Airways jet lag advisor [10] can help individuals plan light and melatonin exposure including in preparation for travel.

7. How do patients generally respond to treatment? What other considerations exist for patients with circadian rhythm disorders?

Treatment of circadian rhythm sleep wake disorders can often be challenging, and requires an individualized and multimodal approach, incorporating behavioral strategies such as directed light exposure, and appropriately timed melatonin. Overall effectiveness can be improved by combining these measures with chronotherapy, which gradually and progressively shifts the circadian clock.

Patients tend to respond well initially, however often require significant personal investment to maintain their newly desired schedule, and relapse to prior sleep schedule is not uncommon. It is essential to have the support of family, friends, teachers and coworkers to establish and maintain a sustainable new sleeping schedule.

When treating circadian rhythm sleep wake disorders, it is important to optimize the treatment of other comorbid medical conditions, especially psychiatric and mood disorders. This is especially true in adolescents and older patients. The importance of addressing sleep hygiene and one's sleep environment cannot be overstated as a critical component of treatment.

The treatment of CRSWDs remain a challenge, in part because of the scarcity of large, multicenter placebo-controlled trials using phototherapy and pharmacotherapy. However there have been recent rapid advances in our understanding of the genetics of circadian rhythm regulation, which may lead to improved diagnostic tools and treatments. For example, technology involving DNA manipulation has been used to generate Cry1/Cry2 knockout animals to further study the expression of specific genes on circadian function [11]. This opens up avenue for new therapeutic approaches in many disorders, specifically neuropsychiatric conditions, associated with circadian rhythm disturbance.

8. Conclusions

Circadian rhythm disorders are common conditions that occur as a result of misalignment between an individual's intrinsic time-keeping system, and extrinsic cues. There are usually multifactorial contributions, including genetic influences, and behaviorally induced elements. Effective treatment approaches largely revolve around strategically timed melatonin and phototherapy to shift one's sleep phase to a more desired time. Consultation with a sleep medicine clinician may be helpful if symptoms persist, or to clarify a suspected circadian rhythm disorder.

Acknowledgements

The authors wish to acknowledge faculty at the Northwestern University Center for Circadian & Sleep Medicine, and the UCLA Sleep Disorders Center for their significant contributions towards our training and sleep medicine education.

Author details

Ajay Sampat[1]* and Armand Ryden[2]

1 UC Davis Department of Neurology, Sacramento, CA, USA

2 VA Greater Los Angeles Healthcare System, Los Angeles, CA, USA

*Address all correspondence to: acsampat@ucdavis.edu

References

[1] Zee PC, Attarian H, Videnovic A. Circadian Rhythm Abnormalities. Continuum (Minneap Minn). 2013 Feb;19(1 Sleep Disorders): 132-47

[2] Reid KJ, Zee PC. Circadian rhythm sleep disorders. Handb Clin Neurol 2011;99: 963-977

[3] Barion A, Zee PC. A clinical approach to circadian rhythm sleep disorders. Sleep Med. 2007 Sep;8(6):566-77

[4] Bjorvatn B, Pallesen S. A practical approach to circadian rhythm sleep disorders. Sleep Med Rev 2009;13(1):47-60

[5] Dodson ER, Zee PC. Therapeutics for circadian rhythm sleep disorders. Sleep Med Clin 2010;5(4):701-715

[6] American Academy of Sleep Medicine. International Classification of Sleep Disorders. 3rd ed. Darien, IL: American Academy of Sleepy Medicine; 2014.

[7] Uchiyama M, Lockley SW. Non–24-Hour Sleep–Wake Syndrome in Sighted and Blind Patients. Sleep Medicine Clinics 2009; 4(2): 195 – 211.

[8] Kolla BP, Auger RR. Jet lag and shift work sleep disorders: how to help reset the internal clock. Cleve Clin J Med 2011;78(10): 675-684

[9] Morgenthaler TI, Lee-Chiong T, Alessi C, et al. Practice parameters for the clinical evaluation and treatment of circadian rhythm sleep disorders. An American Academy of Sleep Medicine report. Sleep 2007;30(11):1445-1459

[10] British Airways Jet Lag Advisor. (2021, June 15). Retrieved from https://www.britishairways.com/travel/drsleep/public/en_gb

[11] Palm D, Uzoni A, Simon F, et al. Evolutionary conservations, changes of circadian rhythms and their effect on circadian disturbances and therapeutic approaches. Neuroscience & Biobehavioral Reviews 2021; Sep 2021 128(21-34).

Chapter 9

Sleep Disorders in Pregnancy

Patrizia Moretti, Giulia Menculini and Lucia Gonfia

Abstract

Sleep disturbances and changes in circadian rhythms are commonly observed in pregnant women. These disorders can result from anatomical, physiological, psychological, and hormonal alterations that can influence sleeping during this phase. Sleep disorders during pregnancy can be responsible for detrimental effects on both mother and foetus. In this chapter we will focus on the epidemiology of sleep disorders, physiological sleep mechanisms and their alterations during pregnancy, as well as on risk factors for sleep disorders in pregnancy. We will then focus of the most frequent sleep disorders during pregnancy, also considering eventual adverse implications for both mother and child, prognosis, and possible pharmacological and non-pharmacological treatments.

Keywords: Circadian Rhythms, Insomnia, Hypersomnia, Sleep disorders

1. Introduction: sleep disorders and changes of circadian rhythms during pregnancy

Sleep architecture and sleep regulation mechanisms are different depending on gender. Indeed, women are used to perceive worse subjective sleep quality when compared to men, as demonstrated by shorter circadian period in this population. Moreover, female tend go to bed earlier and fall asleep later and present a larger melatonin production pattern [1–6]. The prevalence of sleep disorders is also different in males and females. Hence, some disturbances, such as hypersomnia, insomnia, parasomnia, and restless legs syndrome are more frequent in women, while narcolepsy, arousal disorders, Klein-Levine syndrome, and sleep behaviour disorder with rapid eye movement are more frequent in men [7–9].

Pregnancy and perinatal period (one year after childbirth) represent particularly vulnerable periods for women, due to anatomical, hormonal, and psychological changes that infuence women's global health [10]. Poor sleep is a common condition during this period especially during the third trimester [11]. Indeed, 52-61% of women during the last eight weeks of pregnancy show reduced and poor sleep quality, with even higher prevalence among women with a diagnosis of current or previous depressive disorder or history of smoking [7].

Moreover, pre-existing sleep disorders may become more serious during pregnancy and these disturbances increase as the gestational period progresses. Sleep changes in pregnancy are detected by polysomnogram measurements, which during the third trimester usually show an increase in wakefulness after sleep onset and a decrease in Rapid Eye Movement (REM) sleep compared to non-pregnant women [12].

During pregnancy, sleep disorders may contribute to the occurrence of irritability, diurnal hypersomnia with reduction in efficiency, abuse of hypnotic/anxiolytic drugs, impulse control disturbances, also leading to the development of mood

IntechOpen

disorders and to increased suicidal ideation with a risk of suicidal behaviours [12, 13]. Moreover, low birth weight and morphological abnormalities may occur in the foetus and his/her circadian rhythms may also be disrupted, since these are regulated by maternal factors. To note, the foetus does not produce melatonin, a hormone with an essential role in sleep–wake rhythm regulation. Further circadian rhythms that may be altered as consequence of sleep–wake disorders are: body temperature, physical activities, eating patterns, and hormone secretion, particularly melatonin and glucocorticoids These alterations can also explain why pregnant shift-workers display a higher risk of low birth weight, spontaneous abortion, and premature birth, and have sons affected by insomnia or low-birth weight, but also a higher risk of infertility, miscarriage, and pre-eclampsia [7, 13–17].

Previous studies reported different data about the incidence of sleep disorders during pregnancy, but consensus was reached about pregnant women having more disturbed sleep than during other times in their lives. Particularly, about 25% of pregnant women report significant sleep disturbances during the first trimester, with rates rising up to almost 75% during the third trimester [18]. Some authors also argue that up to 97% women report disturbed sleep during pregnancy [19].

2. Factors affecting sleep during pregnancy and action of sexual hormones

Poor sleep quality and insufficient sleep duration are common in the general population and can result from environmental and psychosocial factors, as well as from medical and psychiatric disorders. During pregnancy, possible causes of sleep complaints, such as hormone release alterations, increase their incidence. A relevant role is also played by anatomical and physiological changes.

Sleep disturbances seem to be caused by different factors during the three trimesters of gestation. During the first trimester, the main causes of disturbed sleep are vomiting, nausea, and history of infertility. Gastrointestinal disorders appear to be sleep-disturbing factors also in the second trimester [11], whilst in the last trimester women with muscular-skeletal pain, overweight, restless legs, reflux, uncomfortable positions, and snoring present more sleep disturbances [20].

The main precipitating factors are listed below:

- Anatomical and physiological factors, such as ligament stretching, uterine contractions, or foetal movement;
- Breathing difficulties due to increased uterine volume raising the diaphragm;
- Nocturnal incontinence due to increased sodium excretion during the night;
- Impairment in body movements;
- Hormonal changes, especially ovarian ones;
- Widespread pain and cramps;
- Increased sympathetic nervous system activities;
- Gastrointestinal disorders, such as gastro-oesophageal reflux, constipation, delayed gastric emptyng;
- Anxiety, stress, and tension [10, 21–24] (see **Table 1**).

Pathogenetic factors
- **Socio-demographic**
- age > 30 years old;
- educational level
- single marital status
- history of infertility
- **Psychiatric disorders/symptoms**
- anxiety
- depression
- increased stress level
- predisposing personality traits (internalisation, perfectionism, obsessive, neurotic, and dependent on gratification)
- **hormonal, metabolic and anatomical changes**
- sex hormone fluctuations (increased oestrogen and progesteron, studies about activity of two hormones are still conflicting)
- amplified hypothalamic–pituitary–adrenal axis
- reduced melatonin
- inhibition of the dopaminergic system
- increased prolactin
- nutritional deficiency
- joint pain
- chronic diseases
- cramps
- nausea
- enlarged abdomen and weight gain
- respiratory disorders
- posture restrictions
- nocturia
Pathophysiological consequences of poor sleep quality in pregnant women
- elevate glucocorticoids levels
- oxidative stress
- decreased glucose tolerance
- increased inflammatory cytokines
- dysfunction of serotoninergic system and hyperactivity of noradrenergic system
- deficits in neuroplasticity
- hypertension
Main pathological conditions detected
- psychiatric disorders (anxiety, depression, psychosis and substance or alcohol abuse, suicidal ideation)
- gestational diabetes
- hypertension, pre-eclampsia and eclampsia
- low birth weight and preterm birth
- morphological alterations and foetal disorders
- spontaneous abortion
- increased risk of caesarean section

Table 1.
Overview of the development of new pathological conditions in pregnancy from sleep-altering physio-pathological conditions.

3. Consequences of sleep disorders during pregnancy on women

Sleep is a fine mechanism regulated by different factors and its alteration presents consequences for both the mother and the child. Furthermore, discomfort and frustration experienced by women may also influence their partners, who may in turn present sleep disorders. The most frequent consequences of sleep disorders during pregnancy are discussed in this section.

3.1 Affective disorders and suicidal ideation

Sleep plays a fundamental role in learning, by influencing the development new neuronal circuits. Subsequently, sleep restriction can lead to a disruption of neuroplasticity, thus triggering some among the pathophysiological mechanisms responsible for the development of depression. The pathophysiological mechanisms underlying both sleep disorders and depression are regulated by common neurobiological systems, i.e., hyperactivity of the hypothalamic–pituitary–adrenal axis, dysfunction of serotoninergic system, and hyperactivity of noradrenergic system [25]. Indeed, these specific systems play a role in the regulation of basic emotional responses, such as fear and reward. Therefore, insomnia may compromise adequate emotional processing and may underpin a greater susceptibility to develop psychopathology, particularly anxiety and depressive symptoms and, to a lesser extent, psychosis and substance or alcohol abuse [26].

This may explain why disturbed sleep is reported in up to 90% subjects with depression and REM sleep disturbances may precede the clinical expression of depression itself, aiding the identification of individuals at high risk for developing the disease [27].

However, there are conflicting studies on the correlation between sleep disorders and depression during pregnancy. In previous reports, insomnia did not predict post-partum depression in women with no prior history of depression, as evidenced in a longitudinal study carried out in women at the 17th and 32nd week of gestation and eight weeks after childbirth. This study underlined women suffering from depression before pregnancy also reported more severe residual insomnia symptoms compared to those who scored low for depression at both times [28]. On the contrary, another study showed that poor sleep may represent a potential risk factor for depression during both the prenatal and post-partum period [29]. An Italian study reports that pregnant women with high stress-related sleep reactivity, compared to those with low reactivity, reported more symptoms of insomnia, higher rates of depression, anxiety, and suicidality [13].

Post-partum depression (PPD) is a condition that affects 10-15% of women during pregnancy. It presents with depressive symptoms, such as low mood, hopelessness, sleep disturbances, emotional lability, feelings of guilt, changes in appetite, suicidal ideation, memory loss, fatigue, difficulty in concentrating, and irritability, usually compromising the mother-baby relationship [30]. Physiological, hormonal and metabolic changes occurring during pregnancy often interrupt mother's sleep–wake cycle, and the loss of the sedative effects of endogenous progesterone can lead to post-partum insomnia. In addition, women may wake up several times during the night to take care of their baby and all these factors can contribute to the development of depressive symptoms. Women with a previous history of mood disorders and obsessive–compulsive disorder, as well as women who already presented circadian rhythm disruptions, were also more susceptible to developing this condition. The correlation between sleep disorders and post-partum depression can also be demonstrated by the evidence that treatments for sleep disturbances in pregnant women, i.e. trazodone or diphenhydramine, may contribute to a consequent reduction in symptoms of post-partum depression [12, 30].

Suicidal behaviour is the leading cause of injury and death during pregnancy and suicidal ideation is often considered a key predictor of subsequent suicide attempts [25]. During pregnancy, the prevalence of suicidal ideation can reach between 5 and 14%, which appears to be twice as high as in women without sleep disorders [25, 31]. The presence of comorbid depression leads to a further increase of suicidal risk. Main predisposing factors that lead a pregnant woman to plan suicide are: history of abuse, accidental pregnancy, marital status, family dynamics, low level of education, partner violence, mood disorders, and sleep disorders [25]. The correlation between sleep and suicidal ideation or behaviour can be explained since poor sleep quality may contribute to changes in cognitive, emotional and behavioural processes, and the resulting irritability and emotional lability may encourage suicidal attitude [25, 31].

3.2 Gestational diabetes

Sleep disruptions can exacerbate glucose intolerance. This mechanism can explain why mothers with gestational sleep deprivation during early pregnancy may be up to 4.5 times more likely to develop gestational diabetes than other mothers [32]. Furthermore, mothers with sleep deprivation during pregnancy more frequently give birth to children with a 40% increased risk of overweight and obesity [21].

3.3 Hypertension, pre-eclampsia and eclampsia

Hypertension and pre-eclampsia present an incidence of 5–10% during pregnancy and they can be identified as the main causes of maternal and perinatal morbidity and mortality [33, 34]. Sleep disturbances during pregnancy have been associated with increased gestational weight gain, which can lead to hypertension, pre-eclampsia, and eclampsia [9, 6, 17, 32]. This risk can be even higher during the last trimester, when the increase in oestrogen levels leads to an increase the development of these complications [7].

3.4 Low birth weight and preterm birth

The World Health Organisation (WHO) defines low birth weight (LBW) as a birth weight under 2,500 g, very low birth weight (VLBW) as less than 1,500 g and extremely low birth weight (ELBW) as <1,000. Pre-term delivery is the main cause of perinatal morbidity and mortality. It is also the cause of 75% deaths during childbirth and represents half of long-term neonatal morbidity causes [35]. Reduced maternal sleep duration tends to be associated with lower birth weight [36]. Indeed, LBW incidence appears to be lower among sons/daughters born from women who sleep 9-9.9 hours every night, than among those women sleeping 6-7.9 hours [37]. Sleep deprivation during pregnancy is associated with longer labour during childbirth, lower pain threshold and discomfort, higher caesarean section rates, and preterm delivery [36]. These factors can result from the increase of proinflammatory cytokines, such as interleukin-6, promoting the release of prostaglandins that trigger the onset of labour, thus leading to an increased risk of preterm delivery [36]. This is particularly evident among specific populations, i.e., Afro-American women, that show a risk of pre-term birth increased by 10 times in the presence of sleep disorders when compared to those who have good sleep quality [38]. At the same time, babies who were born prematurely cause concern in new mothers, who will sleep worse and will be more susceptible to postpartum depression [38, 39]. However, further studies on the relationship between sleep and inflammatory markers are needed to better understand their actual correlations [18].

3.5 Morphological alterations and foetal disorders

An association among maternal breathing disorders during sleep and foetal pathologies is already known, but during recent years specific foetal problems also appeared to be associated with other sleep disorders. Indeed. sleep disorders can lead to altered hormone levels, which can activate pathophysiological mechanisms that cause dysfunctions in offspring [40]. Short sleep duration is associated with an exaggerated inflammatory response, i.e., increased circulating and stimulated levels of inflammatory cytokines and sleep disturbances, particularly during the first 20 weeks of pregnancy, may contribute to the activation of inflammatory processes, also by causing stress, which represents a well-known activator of inflammation [16–18]. This hypothesis is based on *in vitro* data, suggesting that an increase in cytokine levels inhibits trophoblast invasion, that would result in subsequent disruption of maternal vascular bed and placental remodelling, an abnormality present in pre-eclampsia, premature birth, and pregnancies with intrauterine growth retardation [18]. Sleep deprivation during the last week of pregnancy caused reductions in the number of nephrons and increased blood pressure in the offspring [41]. Furthermore, gestational sleep deprivation may be associated with an increased risk of overweight and higher blood pressure in offspring up to the age of 11 years, with more pronounced effects in girls than boys [32].

4. Insights into the most common sleep disorders during pregnancy

The following is a description of the most common psychiatric disorders that can be found in pregnant women. Undoubtedly, the most common disorder is insomnia [42], but other disorders such as restless legs syndrome and narcolepsy are should also be considered in order to preserve the health of both mothers and children. Respiratory disorders, such as sleep apnoea syndrome and snoring, may also be encountered during pregnancy [9]; these disorders are not of direct psychiatric interest, but can be differentially diagnosed from other sleep disorders and can sometimes be the cause for these (as in the case of insomnia) and therefore require specialist monitoring [10].

4.1 Insomnia

4.1.1 Definition, predisposing factors and epidemiology

Recent classifications listed in the Diagnostic and Statistical Manual-5th Edition (DSM-5) [43] and in the International Classification of Sleep Disorder- Third Edition (ICSD-3) [44] deleted the distinction between primary and secondary insomnia (that is, dependent on other medical and mental disorders) in favour of a single diagnostic category. Insomnia is defined whether as an independent diagnostic entity or as a comorbidity of other mental, medical, and sleep disorders without the need to establish causal relationships. Spielmann et al. in 1987 proposed the diathesis-stress model of insomnia, which relies on the conceptualisation of the 3P model: predisposing, precipitating and perpetuating factors contribute to the development and maintenance of insomnia [27, 45]. Predisposing factors are already present before the onset of insomnia. Female sex, pre-menstrual syndrome, pregnancy, post-partum, and menopause may influence the risk of developing insomnia. Moreover, reduced melatonin levels, which may be inversely related to gonadotropin secretion, play a relevant role. Anyway, the main of these is represented by sleep vulnerability in response to stress, namely sleeping difficulty due to stressful precipitating stimuli [46]. Furthermore, internalisation, perfectionism, obsessive, neurotic, and dependent personality traits are other factors that may contribute to these effects [47–49]. All this explains particular sleep vulnerability in pregnancy, both because pregnancy itself is a predisposing factor, but also since stress and sex hormones interfere with sleep [16, 17, 50]. Among precipitating factors, there are mechanisms that promote higher likelihood of developing sleep disorders, thus determining the transition from pre-morbid insomnia to acute insomnia. If these disturbing factors are not eliminated, early insomnia may evolve into a chronic form. The main among these precipitating factors are: stress, health problems, pain, anxiety, mood lowering [45].

Insomnia in pregnancy has a prevalence from 5–38% of women in early pregnancy, and it is reported as high as 60% in the eight weeks before the childbirth [7, 9]. Pregnancy is a period characterised by worries, fears and doubts about the health of the baby and this can be a precipitating factor of insomnia as well. As for perpetuating factors, these are mainly represented by behavioural, cognitive and physiological factors that persist in subjects already presenting with insomnia and may lead to chronic insomnia in 80% cases, such as drinking caffeinated beverages in the evening or engaging in stressful activities while lying in bed [45, 51]. Pregnant women with predisposing factors for insomnia and some neuroendocrine alterations can develop precipitating factors, increasing both inflammation modulating factors and amplifying hypothalamic–pituitary–adrenal axis with activation of allostatic load that can cause adverse pregnancy outcomes [16, 17]. Sleep also plays a fundamental role in learning through new neuronal circuits development, and sleep restriction can thus lead to a disruption of neuroplasticity and to the development of the pathological mechanism of depression, given the correlation between the two systems. Therefore, insomnia may compromise adequate emotional processing and may predispose to greater susceptibility to the development of psychiatric symptoms, such as anxiety, depression and, to a lesser extent, psychosis and substance or alcohol abuse [26].

Insomnia in pregnancy can be differentially diagnosed with various disorders that may in turn be comorbidities, causes or consequences of insomnia. The adequate identification of insomnia, as well as other comorbidities, is crucial in order to. The conditions that may underpin differential diagnosis issues with insomnia are the following: Major Depressive Disorder (MDD); Bipolar Disorder (BD); Generalised Anxiety Disorder (GAD); Post-Traumatic Stress Disorder (PTSD); Panic Disorder (PD); Obsessive Compulsive Disorder (OCD); Obstructive Sleep Apnea-Hypopnea (OSAH); Restless Leg Syndrome (RLS) [42].

4.1.2 Pathophysiological mechanisms underlying the development of insomnia during pregnancy

Hormonal changes are the most important factors influencing duration, quality, and physiology of sleep. The action of sex hormones in sleep could be observed in preclinical studies conducted on ovariectomised rats [52]. Steroid hormones, namely oestrogen and progesterone, increase during pregnancy with different and often complementary effects on sleep and respiratory physiology. The early increase in progesterone during the first trimester improves slow-wave sleep and activity through induction of GABA receptors. Indeed, allopregnanolone, a metabolite of progesterone, is a strong modulator of the GABA-A receptor and produces sedative and anxiolytic effects. Progesterone acts as a stimulant of the respiratory drive, as in obese women, increasing the activity of the genioglossus muscle, thereby dilating the diameter of the upper airways. Counterpart to this protective effect against obstructive sleep apnoea (OSA) may be an increased risk of central apnoea, due to hormone-induced re-setting of chemoreceptors that favours hyperventilation/hypocapnia coupling, as well as an increased pressor response to hypercapnia and apnoea [10, 23, 53, 54]. Literature shows that high levels of oestrogens promote sleep [55]. At the same time, some studies report that during the luteal phase of the menstrual cycle (the phase where progesterone levels evidently increase) some women may experience worse sleep [56, 57]. Low levels of oestradiol (E2) due, for example, to lower ovarian production, are associated with worst sleep quality and higher prevalence of insomnia [58]. Studies in rats that were administered oestradiol after sleep deprivation have shown variable results, as sleep worsened according to some authors, while according to others sleep recovery could be facilitated [59]. In postmenopausal women that were given hormone replacement therapy with oestrogen, a subjective improvement in sleep was detected, whether oestrogen was administered orally or transdermal, or when combined with progestin [60, 61]. Different results from several reports may be consequence of a different individual sleep responses to sex hormones activities [55].

4.1.3 Treatment for insomnia

For ethical reasons, investigational drugs are never tested on pregnant women and literature focused on treatments for this population is scant. However, some reports seem to provide preliminary answers. Approximately 1% of women use melatonin during pregnancy. Melatonin is not monitored by the Food and Drug Administration and therefore doses and timing of administration are not well-known or regulated yet [62, 63]. Maternal melatonin is required to synchronise foetal circadian rhythms, but an alteration in endogenous production, including external administration, could alter the amount of melatonin receptors in the foetus. In fact, clinical studies on its use during pregnancy are inconclusive and conflicting [64] Some studies show that melatonin does not cause adverse effects in the offspring and it and may have a protective activity due to its antioxidant properties. Particularly, a study conducted in 2016 showed that prenatal treatment with melatonin significantly reduced neonatal biometry and birth weight [65]. In addition, melatonin treatment increased the duration of gestation by 7.5% and shifted childbirth time, also reducing glucose tolerance and altering hormone levels [19]. Subsequently, the use of melatonin in pregnancy is currently discouraged until more reliable data are available [63]. Although there are concerns about the administration of exogenous melatonin in pregnancy and its impact on the development of circadian rhythms and reproductive function in offspring, exogenous melatonin may also have some potential protective effects on the foetus [9].

Among the drugs most safely used in pregnancy antihistamines are listed, which are used by 10-15% of pregnant women for nausea and vomiting, and which also present sedative effects, so these properties seem to be useful for insomnia treatment [10, 63]. Trazodone can also be proposed as a sedative drug during pregnancy [10, 30] since some studies exclude an association with congenital malformations, although literature is limited [42]. Sedative-hypnotics such as zolpidem have limited data on reproductive safety and therefore their use in pregnancy is limited [33]. However, benzodiazepines can be considered for treatment during pregnancy, taking into account the risk/benefit ratio [9, 42].

Insomnia can be treated both with medication and non-pharmacological treatments. Short-duration and self-limited conditions may not need to be treated, whilst if the disorders are debilitating, it is necessary to assess maternal or foetal adverse effects and impact on quality of life [9].

Pregnant women are reluctant to the assumption of drugs, due to the fear of adverse events on the foetus. For these reasons, women are willing to accept non-pharmacological treatments such as cognitive behavioural therapy (CBT), for which promising results are demonstrated [66, 67]. Further non-pharmacological interventions, such as sleep restriction, stimulus control, relaxation techniques, sleep hygiene and sleep education led to a subjective improvement in sleep quality as well as subclinical anxiety and depressive symptoms [9].

4.2 Disorders of circadian sleep–wake rhythms in pregnancy

4.2.1 Definition and prevalence

According to DSM-5, the diagnostic criteria for circadian sleep–wake rhythm disorders are: persistent or recurrent pattern of sleep disruption due mainly to an alteration of the circadian system or a mismatch between endogenous circadian rhythm and the sleep–wake rhythm required by an individual's physical condition or imposed by social or work commitments; sleep disruption leads to excessive sleepiness, insomnia or both and sleep disruption causes clinically significant distress or impaired functioning in cognitive, social, occupational or other important areas. The prevalence of circadian rhythms disorders is about 3-10% [68].

4.2.2 Pathophysiological mechanisms of circadian sleep–wake rhythm disorders in pregnancy.

Circadian rhythms that may be altered as consequence of sleep–wake disorders are: body temperature, physical activities, eating patterns, melatonin and glucocorticoids secretion [14]. The activation of this system occurs through the action of light, which activates photoreceptive cells in the retina that produce melanopsin and through the retino-hypothalamic tract projected to the suprachiasmatic nucleus of the hypothalamus, regulating various pathways. Alterations in circadian rhythms are known to occur in depressed patients. Indeed, this population of subjects can present abnormalities in the secretion of cortisol, TSH and melatonin, as well as increased internal body temperature at night. Furthermore, there is a clear worsening of depressive symptoms with darkness, which may be clearly evident in seasonal affective disorder, as light therapy is effective in circadian rhythms disorder and SAD [14, 69, 70]. Of particular importance is the interaction between maternal melatonin and glucocorticoid secretion and effects in the foetus [71], as melatonin has a pleiotropic biological action with consequent antioxidant, antidepressant, antihypertensive, epigenetic, and trophic effects on the foetus [72, 73]. At the same time, increased cortisol leads to elevated levels of glucocorticoids and if these are excessive could interfere with foetal tissue [74].

4.2.3 Main clinical manifestations in pregnancy.

Pregnant women may also be affected by circadian rhythms disorders and in this case, in addition to the mood disorders mentioned above, they may present with other pathological conditions and the effects of these alterations are clearly evident in shift workers, who have a higher risk of low birth weight, spontaneous abortion and premature birth, but also a higher risk of infertility, miscarriage, pre-eclampsia [7, 14, 15]. In pregnant rats subjected to altered sleep–wake rhythms an increase of adiposity may occur, together with impaired glucose tolerance, and insulin resistance manifesting in offspring 12 months later [75].

4.2.4 Treatment

In this care, treatment is purely non-pharmacological, based on a correct sleep/wake pattern and bright light therapy [7], but there are still doubts about the actual beneficial effects of this therapy in adult offspring; effectiveness of alternative therapies such as: phytotherapy, acupuncture, acupressure, aromatherapy, reflexology, music therapy and yoga are unknown [71].

4.3 Restless legs syndrome

4.3.1 Definition and epidemiology

Restless legs syndrome (RLS) or Willis-Ekbom disease is a motor-sensory disorder of the lower limbs associated with increased likelihood of sleep–wake disorders, such as poor sleep, poor daytime function and excessive daytime sleepiness in pregnancy. This condition is almost twice as common in women as in men, but reasons for this imbalance in prevalence are not precisely understood [76]. Indeed, the first known epidemiological study of RLS during pregnancy reported a prevalence of 11.3%, but in the third trimester prevalence appeared to rise up to 30%. Pregnancy is a cause of a transitory form of the syndrome, but after several pregnancies it can also become persistent [10].

4.3.2 Pathophysiological Mechanisms.

The main mechanism involved in the pathogenesis of restless legs syndrome is a dysregulation of the dopaminergic system, so a reduction in the absorption of this neurotransmitter favours the development of the disease. In general, pathogenetic factors facilitating the appearance of RLS during pregnancy appear to be:

- Elevate levels of oestrogen, (especially oestradiol, particularly in the third trimester of pregnancy)
- Increased prolactin (decreased action of dopamine)
- Iron-deficiency- related anaemia (common disorder in pregnancy)
- Hypertension (bidirectional relationship) [7, 77, 78].

4.3.3 Treatment

In pregnancy, a correct treatment for RLS can be iron supplementation when needed. Other pharmacological agents, such as clonazepam, clonidine, and opioids may be needed in severe conditions, despite there is a high risk of neonatal withdrawal with these drugs [9, 18]. Non-pharmacological treatments that can be used in pregnant women with RLS are physical exercise and behavioural strategies, such as reduced caffeine intake [76].

4.4 Narcolepsy

4.4.1 Definition epidemiology, pathogenesis

Narcolepsy is a sleep disorder characterised by excessive sleepiness, associated with cataplexy, sleep paralysis, and hypnagogic hallucinations [79]. The prevalence

DOI: http://dx.doi.org/10.5772/intechopen.100300

Disorder	Prevalence	Risk factors	Clinical features	Drug treatments	Non-pharmacological treatments
Insomnia	5–38% of women in early pregnancy, 60% in the eight weeks before childbirth	• Pre-existing predisposing factors • Hormone changes • Physical pathologies • Psychiatric pathologies	• Hypersomnia during the day • Irritability • Mood deflection • Anxiety disorders • Dysregulation of hypothalamic–pituitary–adrenal axis • Excessive inflammatory activation	• Benzodiazepines (selected cases) • Trazodone (assessing risks and benefits) • Difenidramine (assessing risks and benefits) • Melatonin (uncertain)	• Cognitive behavioural therapy for insomnia (CBT-I) • Good sleep hygiene
Restless legs syndrome	11.3% (up to 30% in third trimester)	• Iron deficiency • High levels of oestrogen	• Motor sensory-disorder	• Iron supplements	• Exercise • Reducing caffeine intake
Disorders of circadian rhythms in pregnancy	3-10%	• Alterations in sleep phases • Shift work • Impaired secretion of melatonin and glucocorticoids	• Hypersomnia during the day • Low birth weight • Spontaneous abortion • Premature birth • Sons affected by insomnia • Miscarriage • Pre-eclampsia • Impaired glucose tolerance	• Not recommended	• Correct sleep/wake • Light therapy pattern and bright
Narcolepsy	14/10000 (such as general population)	• Pre-existing disorder • Deficit reticular activating system (RAS)	• Excessive sleepiness • Cataplex • Sleep paralysis • Hypnagogic hallucinations	• Fluoxetine (uncertain)	• Regular naps

Table 2.
Summary of major sleep disorders during pregnancy.

of narcolepsy in the general population is 14/1,000 inhabitants and in pregnant women a similar prevalence can be described. Under a pathogenetic point of view, narcolepsy is the result of an alteration of the nuclei of the reticular system (SRA) that promote wakefulness [7, 80].

Narcolepsy in pregnancy causes adverse effects such as excessive maternal weight gain and gestational diabetes, whilst cataplexy contributes to a higher risk of emergency caesarean section [9].

4.4.2 Treatment

Narcolepsy is less common in pregnancy than other sleep disorders, but is more difficult to manage during pregnancy and in the perinatal period, also due to possible adverse effects of the drugs that may be used. In fact, amphetamines can cause low birth weight and increased risk of miscarriage is reported in women using sodium oxybate [7, 9, 81]. Data on the safety of selective serotonin reuptake inhibitors are conflicting, since there are not significant association with birth defects with use of fluoxetine, but it may contribute to transient neonatal complications during the third-trimester and to risk of social-behavioural abnormalities in childhood [82]. Subsequently, non-pharmacological treatment options are recommended, such as avoiding drugs can cause daytime sleepiness, intermittent napping and practising good sleep hygiene [9] (See **Table 2**).

5. Conclusions

According to Immanuel Kant, 'Heaven has given man three things to compensate for the difficulties of life: hope, sleep and a smile'. Indeed, hope and a smile can also be a consequence of satisfactory sleep, especially during pregnancy, but physical changes and conflicting emotions during this period can at the same time alter sleep patterns. Paying attention to sleep disorders during pregnancy could prevent the development of serious health consequences both for the health of mother and child. Identifying sleep disorders also encourages their adequate and early treatment, thus preventing the development of general symptoms such as asthenia, irritability, and emotional lability, or more serious psychiatric disorders, such as depression, mania and psychosis. At the same time, a multidisciplinary approach to sleep disorders in pregnancy is required. Indeed, the cooperation of psychiatrists, neurologists, gynaecologists, and psychologists may allow a improved sleep quality and increase overall well-being of women, children, and their family.

Author details

Patrizia Moretti*, Giulia Menculini and Lucia Gonfia
Università degli studi di Perugia, Perugia, Italy

*Address all correspondence to: patrizia.moretti@unipg.it

References

[1] Adan A, Natale V. *Gender differences in morningness-eveningness preference*. Chronobiol Int. 2002 Jul;19(4):709-720. doi: 10.1081/cbi-120005390. PMID: 12182498.

[2] Bailey M, Silver R. *Sex differences in circadian timing systems: implications for disease*. Front Neuroendocrinol. 2014 Jan;35(1):111-39. doi: 10.1016/j.yfrne. 2013.11.003. Epub 2013 Nov 25. PMID: 24287074; PMCID: PMC4041593.

[3] Cain SW, Dennison CF, Zeitzer JM, Guzik AM, Khalsa SB, Santhi N, Schoen MW, Czeisler CA, Duffy JF. Sex *differences in phase angle of entrainment and melatonin amplitude in humans. J* Biol Rhythms. 2010 Aug;25(4):288-96. doi: 10.1177/0748730410374943. PMID: 20679498; PMCID: PMC3792014.

[4] Duffy JF, Cain SW, Chang AM, Phillips AJ, Münch MY, Gronfier C, Wyatt JK, Dijk DJ, Wright KP Jr., Czeisler CA. *Sex difference in the near-24-hour intrinsic period of the human circadian timing system*. Proc Natl Acad Sci U S A. 2011 Sep 13;108 Suppl 3(Suppl 3):15602-8. doi: 10.1073/pnas.1010666108. Epub 2011 May 2. PMID: 21536890; PMCID: PMC3176605.

[5] Tonetti L, Fabbri M, Natale V. *Sex difference in sleep-time preference and sleep need: a cross-sectional survey among Italian pre-adolescents, adolescents, and adults*. Chronobiol Int. 2008; Sep25(5):745-759. doi: 10.1080/07420520802394191. PMID: 18780201.

[6] Roenneberg T, Kuehnle T, Juda M, Kantermann T, Allebrandt K, Gordijn M, Merrow M. Epidemiology of the human circadian clock. Sleep Med Rev. 2007 Dec;11(6):429-38. doi: 10.1016/j.smrv.2007.07.005. Epub 2007 Nov 1. PMID: 17936039

[7] Abbott M, Attarian H, Phyllis C. Zee, *Sleep disorders in perinatal women*. Best Practice & Research Clinical Obstetrics & Gynaecology. 2014;**28**(1):159-168 ISSN 1521-6934

[8] Krishnan V, Collop N. *A Gender differences in sleep disorders, Current Opinion in Pulmonary Medicine*: November 2006 - Volume 12 - Issue 6 - p 383-389 doi: 10.1097/01.mcp.00002457 05.69440.6a

[9] Miller MA, Mehta N, Clark-Bilodeau C, Bourjeily G. Sleep Pharmacotherapy for Common Sleep Disorders in Pregnancy and Lactation. Chest. 2020 Jan;157(1):184-197. doi: 10.1016/j.chest.2019.09.026. Epub 2019 Oct 14. PMID: 31622589; PMCID: PMC6965691.

[10] Silvestri R, Aricò I. Sleep disorders in pregnancy. Sleep Sci. 2019 Jul-Sep;12(3):232-239. doi: 10.5935/1984-0063.20190098. PMID: 31890101; PMCID: PMC6932848.

[11] Zhang H. Li P, Fan D, Zhen Wu S., Rao J, Lin D., Huang O., Liu Z. *Prevalence of and Risk Factors for Poor Sleep During Different Trimesters of Pregnancy Among Women in China: A Cross-Sectional Study* Nat Sci Sleep. 2021; 13: 811-820. Published online 2021 Jun 17. doi: 10.2147/NSS.S303763

[12] Obeysekare JL, Cohen ZL, Coles ME, et al. *Delayed sleep timing and circadian rhythms in pregnancy and transdiagnostic symptoms associated with postpartum depression*. Transl Psychiatry. 2020;**10**:14 https://doi.org/10.1038/s41398-020-0683-

[13] Palagini L, Cipollone G, Masci I, Novi M, Caruso D, Kalmbach DA, et al. *Stress-related sleep reactivity is associated with insomnia, psychopathology and suicidality in pregnant women: preliminary results*. Sleep Med. 2019; Apr;**56**:145-150. DOI: 10.1016/j.sleep.

2019.01.009 Epub 2019 Jan 21. PMID: 30803833

[14] Logan RW, McClung CA. *Rhythms of life: circadian disruption and brain disorders across the lifespan*. Nat Rev. Neurosci. 2019 Jan;20(1):49-65. doi: 10.1038/s41583-018-0088-y. PMID: 30459365; PMCID: PMC6338075.

[15] Lyu J, Ye X, Chen Y, Xia Y, Zhu J, Tong S, Yin Y, Qu J, Li S. Children's Sleep May Depend on Maternal *Sleep Duration During Pregnancy: A Retrospective Study.* Nat Sci Sleep. 2020 Mar;10;12:197-207. doi: 10.2147/NSS.S239001. PMID: 32210651; PMCID: PMC7071877.

[16] Palagini L, Biber K, Riemann D. *The genetics of insomnia--evidence for epigenetic mechanisms?* Sleep Med Rev. 2014a; Jun;**18**(3):225-235. DOI: 10.1016/j.smrv.2013.05.002 Epub 2013 Aug 7. PMID: 23932332

[17] Palagini L, Gemignani A, Banti S, Manconi M, Mauri M, Riemann D. Chronic sleep loss during pregnancy as a determinant of stress: impact on pregnancy outcome. Sleep Med. 2014b;**15**(8):853-859. DOI: 10.1016/j.sleep.2014.02.013 Epub 2014 May 27. PMID: 24994566

[18] Okun ML, Schetter CD, Glynn LM. *Poor sleep quality is associated with preterm birth*. Sleep. 2011 Nov 1;34(11): 1493-8. doi: 10.5665/sleep.1384. PMID: 22043120; PMCID: PMC3198204.

[19] Nodine, Matthews *Common sleep disorders: management strategies and pregnancy outcomes J* Midwifery Womens Health, 58 (4) (2013), pp. 368-377.

[20] Sedov ID, Cameron EE, Madigan S, Tomfohr-Madsen LM. *Sleep quality during pregnancy: A meta-analysis*. Sleep Med Rev. 2018 Apr;**38**:168-176. DOI: 10.1016/j.smrv.2017.06.005 Epub 2017 Jun 15. PMID: 28866020

[21] Ferraro ZM, Chaput JP, Gruslin A, Adamo KB. *The potential value of sleep hygiene for a healthy pregnancy: a brief review.* ISRN Family Med. 2014 Feb 17;2014: 928293. doi: 10.1155/2014/928293. PMID: 24967333; PMCID: PMC4041265.

[22] National Sleep Foundation. Sleeping By the trimesters: 1st trimester https://www.sleepfoundation.org/articles/sleeping-trimesters-1st-trimester

[23] Pengo MF, Won CH, Bourjeily G. *Sleep in Women Across the Life Span.* Chest. 2018 Jul;154(1):196-206. doi: 10.1016/j.chest.2018.04.005. Epub 2018 Apr 19. PMID: 29679598; PMCID: PMC6045782.

[24] Wang J, Zhou Y, Qian W, Zhou Y, Han R, Liu Z. *Maternal insomnia during the COVID-19 pandemic: associations with depression and anxiety* Soc Psychiatry Psychiatr Epidemiol. 2021 Apr 23: 1-9. doi: 10.1007/s00127-021-02072-2

[25] Bao C, Xu L, Tang W, Sun S, Zhang W, He J, Zhao K, Xu D, Ye X. *Poor Sleep and Decision-Making Disturbance Are Associated With Suicidal Ideation in Pre-natal Depression.* Front Psychiatry. 2021 May 28; 12:680890. doi: 10.3389/fpsyt.2021.680890. PMID: 34122192; PMCID: PMC8193041.

[26] Hertenstein E, Feige B, Gmeiner T, Kienzler C, Spiegelhalder K, Johann A, et al. *Insomnia as a predictor of mental disorders:* A systematic review and meta-analysis. Sleep Med Rev. 2019;**43**: 96-105. DOI: 10.1016/j.smrv.2018.10.006 Epub 2018 Nov 16. PMID: 30537570

[27] Palagini L, Baglioni C, Ciapparelli A, Gemignani A, Riemann D. *REM sleep dysregulation in depression: state of the art*. Sleep Med Rev. 2013; Oct;**17**(5):377-390. DOI: 10.1016/j.smrv.2012.11.001 Epub 2013 Feb 5. PMID: 23391633

[28] Dørheim SK, Bjorvatn B, Eberhard-Gran M. *Can insomnia in pregnancy predict postpartum depression? A longitudinal, population-based study*.

PLoS One. 2014 Apr 14;9(4):e94674.doi: 10.1371/journal.pone.0094674. PMID: 24732691; PMCID: PMC3986207.

[29] Mellor R, Chua SC, Boyce P. *Antenatal depression: an artefact of sleep disturbance?* Arch Womens Ment Health. 2014;**17**:291-302 https://doi.org/10.1007/s00737-014-0427-6

[30] Khazaie H, Ghadami MR, Knight DC, Emamian F, Tahmasian M. *Insomnia treatment in the third trimester of pregnancy reduces postpartum depression symptoms: a randomised clinical trial*. Psychiatry Res. 2013;**210**(3):901-905. DOI: 10.1016/j.psychres.2013.08.017 Epub 2013 Aug 30. PMID: 23993464

[31] Gelaye, Addae, Neway, Larrabure-Torrealva, Qiu, Stone, Luque Fernandez MA, Sanchez, Williams MA. *Poor sleep quality, antepartum depression and suicidal ideation among pregnant women*. J Affect Disord. 2017 Feb;209: 195-200. doi: 10.1016/j.jad.2016.11.020. Epub 2016 Nov 18. PMID: 27930912; PMCID: PMC5360461.

[32] Harskamp-van Ginkel, Ierodiakonou, Margetaki, Vafeiadi, Karachaliou, Kogevinas, Vrijkotte, Chatzi, *Gestational sleep deprivation is associated with higher offspring body mass index and blood pressure, Sleep*, Volume 43, Issue 12, December 2020, zsaa110, https://doi.org/10.1093/sleep/zsaa110

[33] Bhattacharya S, Campbell DM. The incidence of severe complications of preeclampsia. Hypertension Pregnancy. 2005;24(2):181-90. doi: 10.1081/PRG-200059873. PMID: 16036402.

[34] von Dadelszen P, Menzies JM, Payne B, Magee LA; *PIERS (Pre-eclampsia Integrated Estimate of RiSk) Study Group. Predicting adverse outcomes in women with severe pre-eclampsia*. Semin Perinatol. 2009 Jun;33(3):152-157. doi: 10.1053/j.semperi.2009.02.009. PMID: 19464505.

[35] Goldenberg RL, Culhane JF, Iams JD, Romero R. *Epidemiology and causes of preterm birth*. Lancet. 2008 Jan 5;371(9606):75-84. doi: 10.1016/S0140-6736(08)60074-4. PMID: 18177778; PMCID: PMC7134569.

[36] Warland D. Morrison, O'Brien, *Maternal sleep during pregnancy and poor fetal outcomes: A scoping review of the literature with meta-analysis*. Sleep Medicine Reviews. 2018;**41**:197-219, ISSN 1087-0792 https://doi.org/10.1016/j.smrv.2018.03.004

[37] Murata K. Fukuda, et al. *Maternal sleep duration and neonatal birth weight: the Japan Environment and Children's Study*. BMC Pregnancy Childbirth. 2021;**21**(295) https://doi.org/10.1186/s12884-021-03670-3

[38] Blair P. Leblebicioglu. Christian *Poor sleep quality and associated inflammation predict preterm birth: heightened risk among African Americans Sleep. 2015;38:1259-1267*

[39] Chang JJ, Pien GW, Duntley SP, Macones GA. *Sleep deprivation during pregnancy and maternal and fetal outcomes: is there a relationship*? Sleep Med Rev. 2010 Apr;14(2):107-14. doi: 10.1016/j.smrv.2009.05.001. Epub 2009 Jul 21. PMID: 19625199; PMCID: PMC2824023.

[40] Raimundo JR, Bergamaschi CT, Campos RR, Palma BD, Tufik S, Gomes GN. *Autonomic and Renal Alterations in the Offspring of Sleep-Restricted Mothers During Late Pregnancy*. Clinics (Sao Paulo). 2016 Sep;71(9):521-7. doi: 10.6061/clinics/2016(09)07. PMID: 27652834; PMCID: PMC5004573.

[41] Thomal JT, Palma BD, Ponzio BF, Franco MoC, Zaladek-Gil F, Fortes ZB, et al. *Sleep restriction during pregnancy: hypertension and renal abnormalities in young offspring rats. Sleep.* 2010;33((10)):1357-6.

[42] Hashmi AM, Bhatia SK, Bhatia SK, Khawaja IS. *Insomnia during pregnancy: Diagnosis and Rational Interventions.* Pak J Med Sci. 2016 Jul-Aug;32(4):1030-7. doi: 10.12669/pjms.324.10421. PMID: 27648062; PMCID: PMC5017073.

[43] American Psychiatric Association. *Diagnostic and Statistical Manual of Mental Disorder, DSM-5*. American Psychiatric Publishin, Washington, DC 2012.

[44] American Academy of Sleep Medicine. *ICSD-3-International Classification of Sleep Disorder*. American Academy of Sleep Medicine, Chicago 2014.

[45] Spielman AJ, Caruso LS, Glovinsky PB *A behavioural perspective on insomnia treatment.* Psychiatr Clin North Am. 1987; Dec10(4):541-553. PMID: 3332317.

[46] Kalmbach DA, Cuamatzi-Castelan AS, Tonnu CV, Tran KM, Anderson JR, Roth T, Drake CL. *Hyperarousal and sleep reactivity in insomnia: current insights. Nat* Sci Sleep. 2018 Jul;17;10:193-201. doi: 10.2147/NSS.S138823. PMID: 30046255; PMCID: PMC6054324.

[47] Akram U, Ellis JG, Barclay NL. *Anxiety Mediates the Relationship between Perfectionism and Insomnia Symptoms:* A Longitudinal Study. PLoS One. 2015 Oct 14;10(10): e0138865. doi: 10.1371/journal.pone.0138865. PMID: 26465774; PMCID: PMC4605553.

[48] Brand S, Kirov R, Kalak N, Gerber M, Pühse U, Lemola S, Correll CU, Cortese S, Meyer T, Holsboer-Trachsler E. *Perfectionism related to self-reported insomnia severity, but not when controlled for stress and emotion regulation*. Neuropsychiatr Dis Treat. 2015 Feb;311:263-71. doi: 10.2147/NDT.S74905. PMID: 25678791; PMCID: PMC4322891.

[49] van de Laar M, Verbeek I, Pevernagie D, Aldenkamp A, Overeem S. The role of personality traits in insomnia. Sleep Med Rev. 2010 Feb;**14**(1):61-68. DOI: 10.1016/j.smrv.2009.07.007 Epub 2009 Nov 7. PMID: 19897388

[50] Olcese JM. *Melatonin and Female Reproduction: An Expanding Universe*. Front Endocrinol (Lausanne). 2020 Mar; 6;11:85. doi: 10.3389/fendo.2020.00085. PMID: 32210911; PMCID: PMC7067698.

[51] Riemann D, Nissen C, Palagini L, Otte A, Perlis ML, Spiegelhalder K. *The neurobiology, investigation, and treatment of chronic insomnia*. Lancet Neurol. 2015; May;**14**(5):547-558. DOI: 10.1016/S1474-4422(15)00021-6 Epub 2015 Apr 12. PMID: 25895933

[52] Deurveilher S, Rusak B, Semba K. *Estradiol and progesterone modulate spontaneous sleep patterns and recovery from sleep deprivation in ovariectomized rats*. *Sleep.* 2009;**32**(7):865-877

[53] Baker, Sassoon, Kahan, Palaniappan, Nicholas, Trinder, Colrain *Perceived poor sleep quality in the absence of polysomnographic sleep disturbance in women with severe premenstrual syndrome* J. Sleep Res., 21 (2012), pp. 535-545, 10.1111/j.1365-2869.2012.01007.x

[54] van Broekhoven, T. Bäckström, R.J. Verkes. *Oral progesterone decreases saccadic eye velocity and increases sedation in women* Psychoneuroendocrinology. 2006;**31**(10):1190-1199 ISSN 0306-4530 https://doi.org/10.1016/j.psyneuen.2006.08.007

[55] Morssinkhof MWL, van Wylick DW, Priester-Vink S, van der Werf YD, den Heijer M, van den Heuvel OA, Broekman BFP. *Associations between sex hormones, sleep problems and depression: A systematic review,* Neuroscience & Biobehavioral Reviews, Volume 118,2020, Pages 669-680, ISSN 0149-7634, https://doi.org/10.1016/j.neubiorev.2020.08.006.

[56] Kravitz HM, Janssen I, Santoro N, Bromberger JT, Schocken M, Everson-Rose SA, Karavolos K, Powell LH. *Relationship of day-to-day reproductive hormone levels to sleep in midlife women*. Arch Intern Med. 2005Nov 14 ;165(20):2370-2376. doi: 10.1001/archinte.165.20.2370. PMID: 16287766.

[57] Shechter, P. Lespérance, Ng Ying, N.M.K. Kin, D.B. Boivin *Nocturnal polysomnographic sleep across the menstrual cycle in premenstrual dysphoric disorder* Sleep Med., 13 (2012), pp. 1071-1078, 10.1016/j.sleep.2012.05.012

[58] Kische, Ewert, Fietze, Gross, Wallaschofski, Völzke, Dörr, Nauck, Obst, Beate Stubbe, Penzel, Haring, Sex *Hormones and Sleep in Men and Women From the General Population: A Cross-Sectional Observational Study*, The Journal of Clinical Endocrinology & Metabolism, Volume 101, Issue 11, 1 November 2016, Pages 3968-3977, https://doi.org/10.1210/jc.2016-1832

[59] de Zambotti M, Colrain IM, Baker FC. *Interaction between reproductive hormones and physiological sleep in women*. J Clin Endocrinol Metab. 2015 Apr;100(4):1426-33. doi: 10.1210/jc.2014-3892. Epub 2015 Feb 2. PMID: 25642589; PMCID: PMC4399298.

[60] Donati Sarti, Chiantera, Graziottin, MD; Ognisanti, Ferdinando MD; Sidoli, Cristina MD; Mincigrucci, Parazzini, Gruppo di Studio IperAOGOI *Hormone therapy and sleep quality in women around menopause,* Menopause: September 2005 - Volume 12 - Issue 5 - p 545-551 doi: 10.1097/01.gme.0000172270.70690.5e

[61] Sarti CD, Chiantera A, Graziottin A, Ognisanti F, Sidoli C, Mincigrucci M, Parazzini F; Gruppo di Studio IperAOGOI. *Hormone therapy and sleep quality in women around menopause.* Menopause. 2005 Sep-Oct;12(5):545-51. doi: 10.1097/01.gme.0000172270.70690.5e. Epub 2005 Sep 1. PMID: 16145308.-Sedov ID, Cameron EE, Madigan S, Tomfohr-Madsen LM. *Sleep quality during pregnancy: a meta-analysis. Sleep Med Rev*. 2018; 38:168-176. doi: 10.1016/j.smrv.2017.06.005

[62] Freeman MP, Sosinsky AZ, Moustafa D, Viguera AC, Cohen LS. *Supplement use by women during pregnancy: data from the Massachusetts General Hospital National Pregnancy Registry for Atypical Antipsychotics* Arch Womens Ment Health, 19 (3) (2016), pp. 437-44.

[63] Simriti K. Chaudhry, Leah C. Susser, *Considerations in Treating Insomnia During Pregnancy: A Literature Review,* Psychosomatics, Volume 59, Issue 4, 2018, Pages 341-348, ISSN 0033-3182, https://doi.org/10.1016/j.psym.2018.03.009.

[64] Tamura H, Nakamura Y, Terron MP, Flores LJ, Manchester LC, Tan DX, et al. Melatonin and pregnancy in the human. Reprod Toxicol. 2008 Apr;**25**(3):291-303. DOI: 10.1016/j.reprotox.2008.03.005 Epub 2008 Apr 1. PMID: 18485664

[65] González-Candia A, Veliz M, Araya C, Quezada S, Ebensperger G, Serón-Ferré M, Reyes RV, Llanos AJ, Herrera EA. *Potential adverse effects of antenatal melatonin as a treatment for intrauterine growth restriction: findings in pregnant sheep.* Am J Obstet Gynecol. 2016 Aug;215(2):245.e1-7. doi: 10.1016/j.ajog.2016.02.040. Epub 2016 Feb 20. PMID: 26902986.

[66] Felder JN, Epel ES, Neuhaus J, Krystal AD, Prather AA. *Efficacy of Digital Cognitive Behavioural Therapy for the Treatment of Insomnia Symptoms Among Pregnant Women: A Randomised Clinical Trial.* JAMA Psychiatry. 2020 May 1;77(5):484-492. doi: 10.1001/jamapsychiatry.2019.4491. Erratum in: JAMA Psychiatry. 2020 Jul 1;77(7):768. PMID: 31968068; PMCID: PMC6990703.

[67] Manber R, Bei B, Simpson N. *Cognitive behavioural therapy for prenatal*

insomnia: a randomised controlled trial. *Obstet Gynecol*. 2019;**133**(5):911-919

[68] Kim JH, Duffy JF. Circadian Rhythm Sleep–Wake Disorders in Older Adults. Sleep Med Clin. 2018 Mar;**13**(1):39-50. DOI: 10.1016/j.jsmc.2017.09.004 Epub 2017 Nov 27. PMID: 29412982

[69] Menculini G, Verdolini N, Murru A, Pacchiarotti I, Volpe U, Cervino A, et al. *Depressive mood and circadian rhythms disturbances as outcomes of seasonal affective disorder treatment: A systematic review*. J Affect Disord. 2018;**241**:608-626. DOI: 10.1016/j.jad.2018.08.071 Epub 2018 Aug 15. PMID: 30172213

[70] Monteleone P, Martiadis V, Maj M. *Circadian rhythms and treatment implications in depression*. Prog Neuropsychopharmacol Biol Psychiatry. 2011; Aug 15;**35**(7):1569-1574. DOI: 10.1016/j.pnpbp.2010.07.028 Epub 2010 Aug 5. PMID: 20691746

[71] Hsu CN, Tain YL. *Light and Circadian Signalling Pathway in Pregnancy: Programming of Adult Health and Disease*. Int J Mol Sci. 2020 Mar 23;21(6):2232. doi: 10.3390/ijms21062232. PMID: 32210175; PMCID: PMC7139376.

[72] Naitoh W. Matsumura, *et* al. *Alteration by maternal pinealectomy of fetal and neonatal melatonin and dopamine D1 receptor binding in the suprachiasmatic nuclei*. Biochem Biophys Res Commun. 1998;**253**(3):850-854

[73] Tain YL, Huang LT, Hsu CN. *Developmental Programming of Adult Disease: Reprogramming by Melatonin?* Int J Mol Sci. 2017 Feb 16;18(2):426. doi: 10.3390/ijms18020426. PMID: 28212315; PMCID: PMC5343960.

[74] Wharfe MD, Mark PJ, Waddell BJ. *Circadian variation in placental and hepatic clock genes in rat pregnancy*. Endocrinology. 2011; Sep;**152**(9):3552-3560. DOI: 10.1210/en.2011-0081 Epub 2011 Jul 19. PMID: 21771885

[75] Varcoe T.J., N. Wight, A. Voultsios, *et al. Chronic phase shifts of the photoperiod throughout pregnancy programs glucose intolerance and insulin resistance in the rat* PLoS One, 6 (2011), p. e18504.

[76] Seeman MV. *Why Are Women Prone to Restless Legs Syndrome?* Int J Environ Res Public Health. 2020 Jan 6;17(1):368. doi: 10.3390/ijerph17010368. PMID: 31935805; PMCID: PMC6981604.

[77] Almeneessie AS, Alyousefi N, Alzahrani M, Alsafi A, Alotaibi R, Olaish AH, Sabr Y, Bahammam AS. *Prevalence of restless legs syndrome among pregnant women*: A case–control study. Ann Thorac Med. 2020 Jan-Mar;15(1): 9-14. doi:10.4103/atm.ATM_206_19. Epub 2020 Jan 2. PMID: 32002041; PMCID: PMC6967142.

[78] Dzaja A, Wehrle R, Lancel M, Pollmächer T. *Elevated estradiol plasma levels in women with restless legs during pregnancy.* Sleep. 2009 Feb;32(2):169-74. doi: 10.1093/sleep/32.2.169. PMID: 19238803; PMCID: PMC2635580.

[79] American Academy of Sleep Medicine. *The international classification of sleep disorders*: diagnostic and coding manual, vol. xviii, American Academy of Sleep Medicine, Westchester, Ill. (2005), p. 297.

[80] Slowik JM, Collen JF, Yow AG. Narcolepsy. 2021 Jul 26. In: StatPearls [Internet]. Treasure Island (FL): StatPearls Publishing; 2021 Jan–. PMID: 29083681.

[81] Thorpy M, Zhao CG, Dauvilliers Y. *Management of narcolepsy during pregnancy*. Sleep Med. 2013; Apr;**14**(4):367-376. DOI: 10.1016/j.sleep.2012.11.021 Epub 2013 Feb 21. PMID: 23433999

[82] Clinical Pharmacology Database Fluoxetine. https://www.elsevier.com/solutions/clinical-pharmacology Elsevier, 2019. Accessed May 10, 2019.